FLYING TO THE MOON

A Mother and Daughter's Journey Through Alzheimer's

Jennifer Blackmore

For my mother and son,
with love and gratitude

Prologue

Little pieces of paper, napkins, envelopes and yellow sticky Post-its filled with scribbled words stare up at me. I wrote these in fleeting, stolen moments of inspiration, desperation and, ultimately, sadness.

Days, weeks and years pass, as these little bursts of light emerge through the wall that safeguards me from the strife that was my marriage and from the anguish of witnessing the ravages of Alzheimer's disease that, fragment by fragment, erased the mind of my beloved mother.

I spread these familiar pieces of paper about my bed again, shuffling them and recalling, "It's all waiting there for you, Jenna Doll," my mother says, encouraging me, helping me to find my way home. I record her words on a 3"x5" scrap of paper.

"The world is your oyster, you know," she tells me late one afternoon, observing my exhaustion from my work and home life. Later that night I write her words on an envelope and place it alongside my bed.

Inscribed on a P.F. Chang napkin, "Your beauty is troubled if it cannot play."

Other notes to self include, "Enjoy her presence and wisdom!" And my favorite, "Mom and I talk brilliant nonsense."

This is our story.

The Announcement

"You know, Jenna, I think I'm losing my mind."

Ivy makes this announcement as we sit in the family room on a Sunday morning watching *Meet the Press*. I see fear and desperation in her eyes as she grips her head with both hands.

I'm not shocked by her announcement, having witnessed my mother's struggles over the past few years. How many times I've watched her get lost in familiar places, forget what she said from one minute to the next, search for a word she is unable to retrieve.

"It's okay, Mom," I respond. "Don't worry. I think I'm losing my mind, too."

Leaning forward, she props her arms on her legs, folds her hands and regards me intently. With a twinkle in her bright blue eyes she smiles and says, "To be honest, I'm tired of it anyway."

We laugh; as we often do these days – it helps us cope.

I am being honest too, when I tell her I think I'm losing my mind. Working full-time while taking care of her, living with a dysfunctional stepfamily and trying to make a bad marriage work has taken its toll. Somehow I've lost myself – and lost my way.

Ivy stares at me for a moment, stands up and puts her skinny arms around me. We stand together for a few minutes, holding each other.

"Doll, let's go out on the town, shall we?" she says with a lively voice.

She loves that phrase. I think it reminds her of more carefree days, and I go along, knowing there is no turning back.

"That sounds like a grand idea, Mom!"

We spend the afternoon at Cauley Square, a historic Florida community in southern Miami-Dade County sprinkled with small cottages hand-built in the 1800s by pioneers.

The cottages have been renovated and converted into antique shops, restaurants and artists' studios. Over the years hurricanes have pummeled these to pieces like matchsticks, but its essence prevails. I feel an affinity with the place, having survived Hurricane Andrew in 1992.

I hold my mother's hand as we stroll through its canopied streets lined with giant ficus trees, Royal Poincianas bursting with fiery red-orange blossoms and pink and red bougainvillea bushes. We step onto the wood porch of the Tea Room and smile at the bas-relief mural covering a wall, a profile of a mother and daughter dressed in turn-of-the-century attire sitting across from each other at a café table, drinking tea. We're reminded of simpler times.

I open the screen door and we walk hand-in-hand into the foyer. An uneven Florida pine floor is covered with Oriental rugs in various sizes and colors. The interior is filled with white wicker furniture, antiques and china plates and trays painted with red, pink and yellow roses lining the walls. Delicate lace curtains cover the windows. It reminds me of trips to my grandmother's house, whom I visited often as a little girl.

Her name was Linnie, but we called her Mammy. Our relationship was sweet and simple, unlike her more complicated relationship with Ivy. When they were together, I rarely sensed a feeling of warmth between them. Mammy had paid for Ivy's two brothers' college education, and I suspect my mother resented having to work for seven years to pay her own way, though she never admitted this.

I used to sit for hours on her living room floor playing with pennies she stored in a jumbo-sized Pond's Cold Cream jar. I loved to turn it upside down and watch dozens of pennies topple out and bounce onto the floor like a miniature waterfall. My little fingers spread them over the carpet with the excitement of an artist putting paint to canvas. I formed all kinds of images with them: horses and cats, circus performers, landscapes with buildings and trees. I created a magical world with those pennies.

Mammy loved to garden and grew rhubarb in her back yard. She baked the most beautiful pies, topped with a pie crust carefully pinched at its edges and adorned with graceful swirls she sliced with a knife. I learned from her how to roll the dough and seal the top and bottom crusts with my forefinger and thumbs. She let me try my hand at the swirls, but mine were no match for hers.

The Tea Room has beautiful pies, too. Whenever Ivy and I go out it feels like a celebration, and this time is no different. We order glasses of chardonnay, quiche, homemade tomato soup and tea sandwiches made with banana nut bread filled with cream cheese and olives. The cooks cut off the crusts the way Ivy used to when she hosted her bridge club parties. Memories of grandmothers, mothers and daughters fill the air with sweetness.

We laugh and put our worries aside, at least for the afternoon.

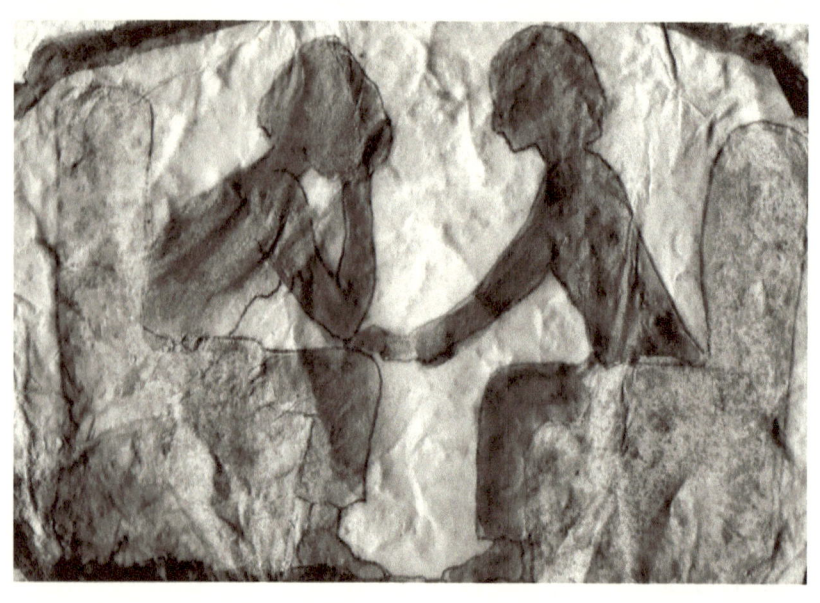

You know, Jenna, I think I'm losing my mind.

The Big House

I am married and part of a blended family of seven. All but my stepson, who is away at college, live here in this house. Mom lives half the year in Columbus, Ohio, staying here in Miami during the winter. She loves our home and calls it *Shangri-La* and "the Land of Milk and Honey." I love it too, and will never forget the first time I saw it.

It was April 1996. My husband Tom and I were newly married, he for his third time, me for my first. We had decided to look for a larger house to accommodate our merged families. He found a unique property in the Redland, an agricultural area southwest of Miami, and arranged for us to see the property the next day.

We drove south for some twenty miles, past nurseries, strawberry farms, ramshackle U-Pick stands, avocado groves and expanses of unspoiled greenery. The house was on a street lined with hardwood trees that formed an uninterrupted canopy overhead.

The driveway, bordered by lush foliage, was positioned at an angle. We pushed the button on the intercom to let the real estate agent know we had arrived, then watched a heavy cedar gate creak slowly to the left, its wheels screeching and lumbering under the weight of its load. We emerged slowly through the entrance onto a serpentine driveway more than 600 feet long that wound its way through an undisturbed landscape of century-old live oaks, palms, bromeliads perched in trees and rooted in the ground, tropical wildflowers, cycads and giant wild Indian tamarind trees. Birds of many species and colors circled above us. We parked the car in front of a guest sign made of rough-sawn cedar. As I walked over Chattahoochee pavers toward the house, my knees started to weaken. I felt protected in this place, a feeling that had escaped me since I married into this stepfamily. I wondered if moving here might change things.

To my left a frangipani tree was in bloom and, adjacent to it, an orange jasmine exploding with delicate white blossoms that belied its powerful scent. I inhaled deeply, now completely intoxicated by the sensuous beauty of my surroundings. As we stepped onto the porch a gumbo limbo tree spared by the architects was growing through the wooden floorboards like a dancing sentinel, its red bark peeling like tissue paper.

As we stepped inside a soft, golden light filtered through the picture windows opposite the foyer and an expansive green vista filled the glass frame. To our right was a massive stone fireplace built of coquina, a limestone composed of crushed shells and coral, each piece strategically placed to create a mosaic of shadows and textures. A plain cedar beam served as a mantel over the hearth. We stood in awe.

We continued the tour, walking on clouds. The five bedrooms and four-and-a-half baths offered plenty of room for our newly blended and extended family. We moved in six weeks later.

Duets

Ivy and I are sitting together at the piano in the living room, the heart of this glorious setting, gazing outside at nature's explosion of beauty. We've lived in the Big House for several years now and I've never really felt safe. Happiness is as fleeting as the butterflies that hover over the honeysuckle bush outside. Ivy and I grab onto whatever makes us happy, like playing duets on the piano.

My mother started lessons at age five and continued until her teacher stated, "I can no longer continue as your teacher. I've taught you everything I know."

She was 15 at the time. Her lessons were a special gift from her mother during the Depression. A disciplined and practical woman, Mammy saw to it that her only daughter practiced every day before school. There were mornings when Ivy, immersed in her music, was late, which wasn't unnoticed by her strict teacher.

"I had to sit in the corner with a dunce cap on my head," she told me. "But even though I felt ashamed, I continued to practice in my mind."

Mammy must have known her daughter's gift would be a way of earning money for the family. At 16 my free-spirited and fun-loving mother formed a band with musical friends and traveled to various clubs around Ohio. Playing by ear, she could transpose keys with ease and eventually landed a job accompanying vocalists on the radio at night. This was the era of Jazz and Blues, an exciting time for a gifted musician. I often heard her say, "During the Depression we didn't have any money, but we had *Song*."

We still have *Song*, sitting side by side at the piano, laughing, singing, talking and losing ourselves in the music, in the moment, like when I was a little girl.

The centerpiece of my childhood home was the Mason and Hamlin concert grand piano that Ivy and my father had purchased at the Capital University School of Music sale. It reigned in our living room next to the tall picture windows, holding court like royalty. When Ivy sat down to play, her music beckoned family and friends to join in the songfest. My sisters and I sometimes spread a blanket beneath the piano and played with our dolls. I remember climbing up one side of the piano and curling into a ball on top of the strings. What Ivy cherished, I also cherished.

I share my mother's musical talent, but am not as confident as she because I didn't practice so much. I enjoyed playing, and often played songs by ear. My first piano teacher frightened me when she slapped my hands if I missed a note. My lessons lasted from age six to 13, until I begged my mother to let me quit. Years later she confessed her ambivalence about the sacrifices she made having to spend most of her childhood and adolescence practicing. During one of our piano fests we talked about it.

"I hated performing, and those recitals were terrifying, Mom."

"That's because I didn't make you practice enough," she said. "I played for a long time, for ten years."

"There's no reason to feel guilty, Mom. You made me practice, but I wasn't confident."

"Jenna Doll, let's play *Fascinatin' Rhythm*," she says. "I love that."

We laugh as our fingers fly across the keys.

"That was a good one!" I say.

She smiles and shakes her head, "Oh, I don't know about that."

We sit for hours at my baby grand piano, reveling in our camaraderie as the pink-orange rays of the sunset wash over us. We live in the moment.

Ten Cents a Dance
That's what they pay me,
Gosh how they weigh me down!

I feel used and weighed down these days, too. We continue to laugh as we play.

Don't know why
There's no sun up in the sky
Stormy weather

The sun shines every day, but its warmth escapes me. We play our hearts out.

They're writing songs of love,
But not for me
A lucky star's above,
But not for me

But not for me either.

The grand finale, also Ivy's signature piece, is Rachmaninoff's *Prelude in C-sharp Minor*. Afterward, I clap and shout, "Bravo!"

"Gee, aren't we rich?" she says with a smile that beams across her face.

"Don't tell anybody."

She leans close to me and whispers in my ear, "They already know."

9

"Guess what, Mom? I recorded you."

I'd placed a tape recorder in the corner of the living room and turned it on when she started to play two hours earlier.

"You, *what?*"

"I recorded you."

"You reported me? Oh no! They found out!"

"I'm afraid the party's over," I tease.

"Jenna, I was afraid the party was over, and I had to hang myself up."

"It's never over, Mom."

As we get up from the piano she adds, "The party isn't over – it's just getting started!"

"On that note," I say, "let's pour ourselves another glass of wine."

The Life Raft

Ivy taught me to appreciate words and poetry as well as music. We made frequent trips to the library when I was a child and, when we returned home, I would spread my armload of books all over the living room floor and devour them.

Before she started losing her mind, she recited her favorite poems often, so much so that I learned many of them just by listening to her.

We spend hours now sitting in our butterfly chairs on the balcony overlooking the treetops with our cat Chris celebrating the beauty of poetry. One of our favorites is *The Highwayman,* by Alfred Noyes.

And still of a winter's night, they say, when the wind is in the trees,
When the moon is a ghostly galleon tossed upon cloudy seas,
When the road is a ribbon of moonlight over the purple moor,
A highwayman comes riding –
Riding – riding
A highwayman comes riding,
Up to the old inn door

An elegant lady with an independent spirit, Ivy walks in short, hurried steps, always with purpose, as if on the verge of making an important announcement.

Most of her friends followed the traditional path of marriage and children right out of high school, but Ivy was determined to get a college degree. She played piano for tuition money and, seven years later, was awarded a degree in Fine Arts from Ohio State University. I have the black-and-white photo of her standing proudly in her cap and gown alongside her mother.

Ivy is a free thinker, but outwardly restrained and proper, her true feelings often buried. I've heard her say time and again, "One must always preserve the amenities, Jenna."

She rarely raised her voice to her children; she didn't have to. If my sisters and I missed the bus and she had to drive us to school, she insisted we make our beds and perform extra chores before taking us. We rarely missed the bus.

She also expected us to face our fears head-on. This was a challenge for a shy child like me, whose fear of the dark and overactive dream life would frequently terrify me.

During the 1950s we lived in a single-story ranch house in what was considered "the country." I loved listening to nature's night sounds, so vast and varied; the soft rustling of leaves brushing against one another in an erratic wind, unidentifiable creatures howling at the moon, the steady drone of cicadas. From my bed I watched the evening sky exploding with stars and a moon whose subtle blue gradations stirred my imagination. Lightning bugs flickered on and off like Christmas tree lights, adding a yellow accent to the midnight blue canvas. The rumble of train wheels in the distance brought fears of hobos somehow making their way to our secluded compound.

I shared a bedroom with my older sister Peggy, providing some degree of comfort. But she had little patience for my wild dreams and irrational fears. So from time to time, I would make my way down the long, narrow corridor to my parents' bedroom. If I awakened Ivy, she would send me right back. My father was more understanding and tolerant, but the lesson was always, "Face your fears, Jenna."

Maintain decorum, keep the peace – this was the code of her era. Another common expression was, *"Sometimes you need to just walk away."*

This I can relate to, especially these days in the Big House – a place inhabited by angry, demanding and judgmental people. I married blindly into this dysfunctional stepfamily, an assemblage of unrelated mothers, fathers, grandmothers and children, a makeshift family in conflict.

When Tom and I met, we were both unattached parents struggling to raise our children. It seemed logical. His daughter and son needed a mother in their daily lives; I was estranged at the time from my son's father, and my eight-year-old son Jonathan needed a man in his life.

At first our relationship seemed promising. I was introduced to Tom by a neighbor who described him as "a regular guy taking care of his kids."

When my neighbor and his wife invited us to dinner, Tom's children, then eight and 14 years old, were with their mother in North Carolina.

He spent the evening ranting about his ex-wife's many shortcomings as a mother. In his mind, I suppose, this boosted his self-image as the *good* parent.

I spent the evening ignoring him, listening to my neighbor's collection of classical CDs, uninterested.

At the end of the evening he said, "Let me walk you home, Jennifer."

Reluctant as I was, I reminded myself to "preserve the amenities."

As we walked the short distance to my townhouse, he picked up Jonathan who immediately pulled away. My son's instincts were clear; I buried mine.

We dated for three years. The children kept busy with sports while Tom and I worked fulltime, but continued living in our separate homes. There was some degree of comfort in the togetherness we felt as a family unit.

I was so touched one evening when Tom's daughter Katie who, like Jonathan, was then 11 years old, knelt before me on one knee and said, "Jennifer, will you marry my dad so I can have a mother and Jonathan can have a father?"

Tom and I married in 1994. The man I married is not who I thought he was.

He can be charming, persuasive and generous. I learned, too late, that his generosity always has strings attached, like strands of hot glue weaving a tangled web that burns badly and for a long time. Early on, his energy was devoted to selling himself to me and to my family. He took us to assorted islands around South Florida on weekend vacations. Once he bought tickets for my entire family to see *Phantom of the Opera*, making a point of giving Jonathan the best seat to prove to everyone, I suppose, what a great stepfather he was. I went along, wanting to believe his magnanimity was genuine. But then the web started to unravel.

When my father passed away two years after Tom and I wed, I was crying in bed, heartbroken. My husband, annoyed because he had to get up early the next morning and wanted to sleep, said, "If you don't stop crying, I'm going to go to a hotel!"

I continued to cry for days, doubly grieved.

Tom's relationship with Jonathan is strained, all trust shattered by his intermittent, irrational outbursts of anger. These continue despite of my protests and attempts to reason. Any fortitude I once felt is now crumbling. I laugh a lot, but feel sick inside. I've turned into a shadow of my former free-spirited self. My husband has somehow overpowered me, and all I foresee is a future fading to a dirty gray.

Once a struggling single mother, independent and in charge of my life, I'm now a used, abused and disrespected third wife, short-order cook and despised stepmother, trying to protect my son and my mother while maintaining my full-time art therapy position with the Miami-Dade County school system. The Big House has turned into a prison inhabited by a dysfunctional family whose secrets, distorted communication and tensions never ease. Nothing I do or say makes a difference.

Ivy watches the show from the sidelines and supports me like a dedicated coach cheering on her prized player. We stand by each other, reluctant actors in a tragic play.

I was brought up in a household where parents and children had mutual respect. But I now realize children have no voice and no rights, according to Tom. Breaking their spirit is "standard procedure."

Tom uses his outbursts of anger to control people and situations. They come on unexpectedly, and I find them frightening. When these run their course he grins like a Cheshire cat. He believes they are justified, and he has self-control because he never hits people; he pummels them instead with his words and fury.

The day of reckoning comes on a Saturday. Jonathan, now 14, adores our two new dogs – Cleo, a black Great Dane, and Patch, a Dalmatian. He feeds them some cans of Purina he finds in our pantry, left by the previous owners of our home. Weeks earlier Tom made an arbitrary decision that they are to be fed only dry food; he often makes nonnegotiable rules, regardless of others' opinions. When he returns from his office to discover that Jonathan fed them the "wrong" food, he explodes.

Ivy and I are sitting on stools in the kitchen, watching our cat Chris in a live oak tree stalking a blue jay gorging at the bird feeder.

One of the advantages of this big rambling house is its ease of isolation. Everyone can hide – both Jonathan and Katie are experts at this. Everyone remains silent and hidden when Tom is home, now prisoners under the watchful eye of a moody and sadistic warden.

I've been a single parent since the day my son was born. Although he and I lived alone for most of his childhood, we're part of a loving family: Mom, Dad, now deceased, my sisters and brother, nieces, nephews and friends. My son and I have always stood by each other, our love and mutual respect unwavering. We both know this stepfamily is nothing like ours.

Jonathan is an even-tempered young man, wise beyond his years. The rage and volatility of his stepfather is alien and unnerving, but he has learned to protect himself by staying quiet and keeping a safe distance.

Ivy and I are jolted out of our reverie by ranting that intensifies as Tom storms into the kitchen, tossing his leather briefcase across the floor.

"Jonathan!" he yells. "Get in here!"

Jonathan runs to the kitchen from the other side of the house, his eyes wide with fear.

"What did I tell you about the dog food?"

Jonathan knows that whatever he says will be blasted out of the air, so his response is reasoned and brief. He chooses his words carefully, but it's as futile as reasoning with a rabid dog.

I stand between them, my chest held high, eyes like daggers, a mother fearless but frightened, desperate and determined to protect her son and defuse her husband's rage.

Tom continues to gesture and flail, spewing venom like the snakes that slither around in our yard.

Ivy has never before witnessed his tantrums. He used to be more controlled in her presence, but what little control he had has now evaporated.

She flees the scene in horror.

When Tom's tirade sputters, I follow Jonathan to his room, my heart pounding.

"I'm so sorry, Jonathan," I say weakly. "You know, Tom has a lot of problems, and they have nothing to do with you and nothing to do with me." I've lost count of the many times I've repeated this mantra. My words sound empty and defeated, a ghost's pleadings, distant, removed and inconsequential.

"I'm fine, Mom," he says with finality, his inner strength and determination trumping any emotional pain or humiliation he feels.

Guilt pours over me like acid rain. I leave Jonathan and go to my mother, now dressed completely in black, as if in mourning. She lies on her bed, shaken.

"I don't know what to say, Mom." My eyes well up with tears. "Are you all right?"

"Of course I'm not *all right*," she responds angrily.

Her lips are parched, and her hands tremble.

"What should I do?"

I'm hanging from a cliff, helpless.

"I can't tell you what to do," she says, her words clipped and razor sharp. They sting.

I take a deep breath and choke on the toxic air that permeates this house.

Minutes later we all flee. Jonathan goes to a friend's house, and I take Ivy to the mall where we walk in silence. She now knows that I married a monster.

The charade continues. We all walk on eggshells, trying to survive. The holidays arrive, which always bring more tension to the Big House, and this year is no exception. We're gathered with family and friends for a Thanksgiving feast, enjoying drinks and hors d'oeuvres by the pool. Cleo breaks out of the dog pen after Jonathan locks her in, jumps on Tom and splashes his shirt with red wine.

He lashes out, "Jonathan, didn't I tell you to lock the dogs in the pen?"

"I did," he says defensively. "Cleo must have jumped against the door and unlatched it. She sometimes does that."

Tom grabs the leash, hooks it on Cleo's collar and yanks her hard. He bolts back to the pen with her in tow, cowering, her lanky frame moving in an awkward, halting gait as she tries to protect herself from his aggression. I hear the gate slam.

The Thanksgiving celebration continues as I sleepwalk through the rest of the day, playing gracious hostess, accomplished cook, pianist, loving mother, sister and daughter, trying valiantly to contain my frayed nerves and boiling rage.

Later that evening as my sister Peggy and I watch the bamboo palm outside sway rhythmically in the breeze, I crouch on the floor next to her as a flood of emotion gushes out, my fragile defenses bruised and broken down. I rock back and forth uncontrollably, choking on words and lack of air.

"A good mother doesn't subject her son to cruelty!" I continue the chant over and over again, trying desperately to release my guilt, anger and sadness. Minutes turn to hours. I continue to rock and sob.

Peggy watches helplessly, fear and concern in her eyes.

"Snap out of it, Doll!" she repeats again and again.

I finally stop and stare at her, empty and dazed.

Still shaking, I stand weakly with Peggy's support. Neither of us knows what to say, so we hug each other and say goodnight.

As the months pass, my marriage continues to spiral out of control. Joining my mother saves me. Artists and Alzheimer's sufferers share a vantage point. Rules are suspended; there are no *should's* or *have to's*. In our upside-down, backward and inside-out world all things nonsensical are celebrated. Seeing the world this way frees us from a frightening and oppressive reality. This new perspective makes sense to us and is definitely more fun – and my mother and I are in this together.

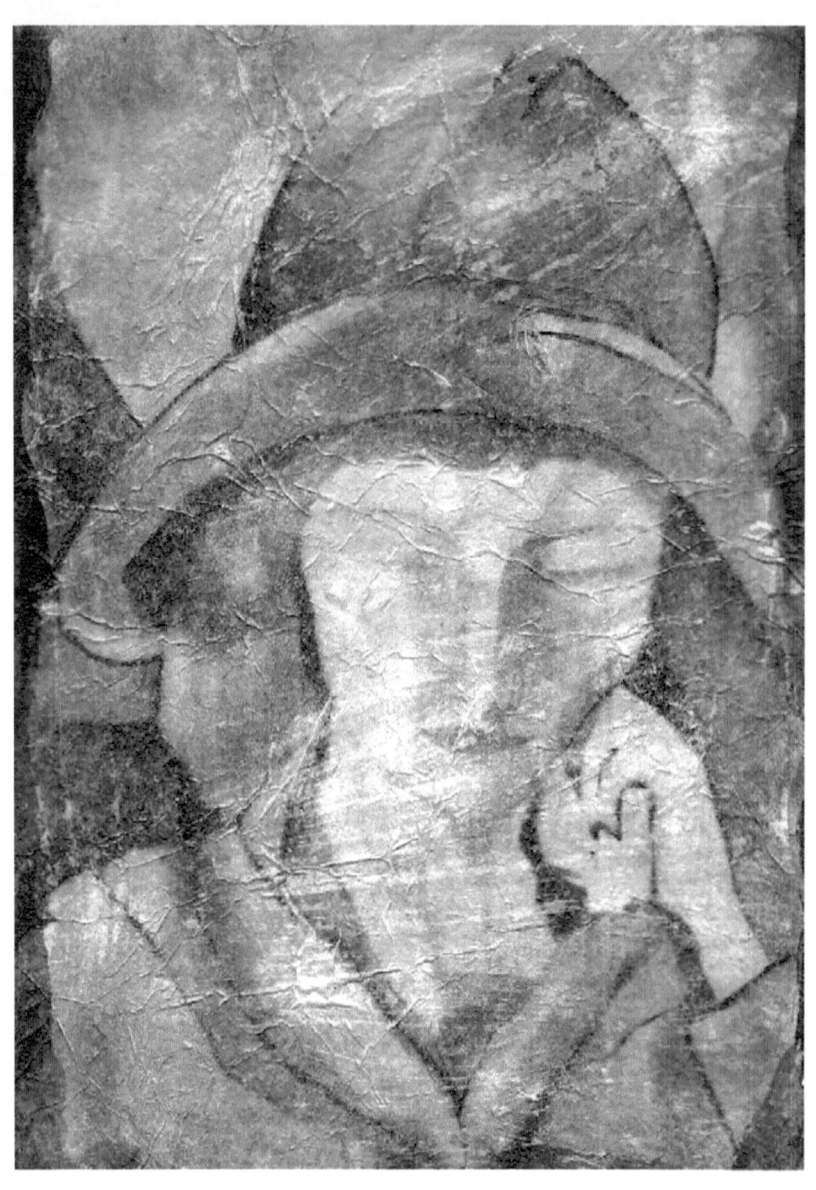

Your beauty is troubled when it cannot play.

Lost and Found

Ivy began to become disoriented, whether walking or driving, when she was still living alone in Ohio. She always made light of it, as though it were an adventure we didn't understand.

"What's all the fuss about?"

It's Saturday afternoon, and we decide to see *Titanic,* the movie now playing at the Falls, a lush, elegantly landscaped Miami mall with shops on either side of streaming waterfalls and one of our favorite destinations. The Falls reminds Ivy of her older brother, a landscape architect, and we share his love of plants.

We sit halfway down, close to the aisle, drink our Sprites and share a small bag of popcorn. Time passes, and I'm captivated. The ship is starting to sink and Leonardo de Caprio and Kate Winslet hang from the bow, preparing for their descent into the dark, frigid waters of the North Atlantic.

"All this water – I have to go to the bathroom."

This is the best part of the movie, and I don't want to leave. A small voice tells me to go with her, but I ignore it.

"Come right back, Mom."

"I'll be all right."

After she leaves, the voice in my head becomes louder. *That was a mistake; you should have gone with her.* I turn to the back of the theater every few seconds waiting for her to reappear. Five minutes pass. The path from apprehension to fear to panic is instantaneous. *I shouldn't have let her go alone. I'm a bad daughter.*

The drumbeat of my heart warns me of impending doom, my mouth turns to sandpaper. I'm not in a movie theater anymore. Feeling the terror of both a toddler separated from Mommy and a mother who has lost her child, I bolt out of the seat and start to search. A teen-aged ticket taker in a red vest jokes with a co-worker as I approach.

With a shaky voice I ask, "Have you seen a small elderly woman dressed in light blue?"

He shakes his head and shrugs his shoulders. "No, sorry."

I circle the lobby, asking anyone in a red vest the same question.

"She sometimes gets confused. She has short white hair and light blue eyes," I ask everyone and nobody.

We had shopped earlier at Chico's, leaving our purchases while we went to the movie. I think that maybe she went back there, confused.

I'm in full panic mode now, thinking *I'm never going to see her again,* but push away that thought as I enter Chico's.

"Did my mother come back here? Remember, we were here about two hours ago?"

"I'm sorry, she didn't. Is everything all right?" I shake my head, and then take the bag containing our purchases and leave.

Fear is beginning to take hold of me as I encounter a security guard, but I'm still coherent enough to tell him what has happened. He asks for a complete description, and I repeat it – twice. He alerts others on his radio while I pace, walk in circles, search, and search some more.

Please be okay, Mommy.

Mall security has alerted the staff at the theater by now, and another ticket taker comes up to me.

"How long has it been since your mother left?"

I somehow find a voice, small and tremulous, like the panicked passengers' voices on the Titanic.

"Um...I don't know, maybe 30 minutes ago." *It seems like five hours.*

"Were you watching *Titanic*?"

"Yes."

"I think I know where she is." He escorts me down the corridor.

"Is that your mother in the doorway over there?"

I see her standing there without a care in the world. I want to scream at her, shake her, punish her, weep, shower her with hugs and kisses – and never let her out of my sight again.

"Mom!" I hug her and grab her hand, tears cascading down my face like the waterfalls outside.

"Is something wrong?"

After leaving the bathroom, she had returned to another screening of the film in a different theater. She hadn't realized she was lost and wasn't afraid; she knew I would find her.

We leave the Falls and return home in silence. My insides are raw.

Everything is different now. I can't trust that she will find her way home. She loves to take long walks around our property. This is a problem. In back are an avocado grove and neighboring horse farm. I have an internal alarm clock now and check on her often.

Some months pass. It's late afternoon on a Saturday, and my instincts warn me of danger.

"Have you seen Grandma, Jonathan?"

"No, not lately."

"Look for her in the avocado grove. I'll drive around in the car."

He jumps up, "Okay, Mom."

Fear tastes familiar now. I start the car and proceed down our long, snaky driveway, clicking the remote that opens our gate. Once comforted by this carefully crafted barrier protecting me from outside danger, I now see prison bars too slow to open as I turn out of the driveway.

I don't see her ahead and make another turn past the brightly colored daycare center, formerly a hardware store. Its colors irritate me. A final turn down the narrow, secluded road behind our property proves fruitful. A half-mile ahead is a vision of blissful eccentricity: Ivy is strolling down the middle of the road, flanked by our dogs, a glass of chardonnay in her right hand. A white ankle sock is on her left foot; a knee-high stocking on her right. I can't help but laugh with relief, as I pull beside her and lower the passenger side window.

"Do you need a lift?" I ask with a smile.

She smiles back, delighted to see me, as though it were happenstance I was driving by.

"Sure, why not?"

Jonathan walks the dogs home through the grove while I drive around the block to the main entrance.

"How was your walk, Mom?"

"Beautiful!"

She's holding a blue jay feather in her hand, a small treasure found on her journey. My pulse and breathing return to normal. Another day, another adventure – how can I be angry with her?

Hidden Treasures

It happened gradually, Ivy putting things in odd places, in strange juxtapositions: a cereal box wrapped in her nightgown, tucked away in the drawer; a half-eaten meal concealed behind her shoes in the corner of her closet; her toothbrush propped in a Kleenex box next to neatly folded white ankle socks – hidden surprises awaiting discovery.

"Mom, what's this?"

My voice is like a lullaby now when I speak to her, a mother interacting with her small child.

I find a croissant in her wine glass.

"How did that get there, Jenna Doll?"

"I don't know – did you put it there?" I say with a smile.

"Who knows?" She shrugs her shoulders and turns her hands up like a mischievous child telling a white lie.

We laugh.

She's aware she is losing her memory and writes her thoughts, cherished poems and fleeting words of wisdom on small pieces of paper, on envelopes and napkins. Her handwriting is shaky, her words misspelled.

Poetry no longer flows easily from her lips. It comes out in bits and spurts, like water making its way through a clogged drain. She has inscribed lines from one of her favorite poems by William Cullen Bryant, *Thanatopsis*, on an envelope embellished with spring flowers and a butterfly:

So live that when thy summons comes to take
Thy? In the sylant? hals of death, thou go not as

My heart feels heavy. I see her desperation and confusion. She used to spell perfectly.

I feel desperate and confused, too. I want to save her. I want to save *both* of us from this foreign and frightening reality.

It's a Sunday afternoon, a perfect time for us to retreat to the corner of our pool deck to escape the tension inside.

Ivy and I cocoon ourselves in our private world. It saves us from absorbing the fury that has taken a permanent hold inside. Hidden treasures save us, providing comic relief. Music and poetry brighten our world. We savor whatever light and happiness we can.

As we sit in our blond teak deck chairs, Chris lounges overhead on the screened enclosure, one leg dangling to the side. We admire the resolve, independence and aloofness of our noble cat.

We listen to the high whistle of leaves and inhale the sweet scent of gardenia blossoms. This is the perfect setting for our poetry fest, and I recite the first line of Edna St. Vincent Millet's *Spring,* another favorite:

"To what purpose, April, do you return again?"

"Remember the next line, Mom? *Beauty...*"

"Beauty..." she hesitates.

"Now it's your turn." This has become a standard response to deflect attention away from memory lapses.

*"Beauty is not...*you know it, Mom.*"*

She concentrates as I wait patiently, resisting the urge to speak for her.

"Beauty is not...enough." She smiles as the words begin to flow.

"You can no longer... you remember, Mom."

"You can no longer quiet me with the redness

Of little leaves opening STICKILY." She loves to enunciate the word STICKILY.

"Beauty is not enough. I know what I know." The last line is spoken with authority.

"Excellent. You remember!"

She beams with pride and says, "You saved me, Doll!"

"*You* did it, Mom!"

Treasured words are recalled, the smallest victories celebrated.

An uncharted reality is closing in on us. I bury my fear and sadness as we continue our poetry fest in its new form and place. I used to follow her; now she follows me. But that's all right. We're not alone.

Temperatures Rising

This is a household at war. It's falling apart at the seams.

Tom's 91-year-old grandmother keeps Ivy company during the day, but any pleasantry she can muster is undermined by unpredictable and explosive tantrums – like grandmother, like grandson. I hear her ranting at the housekeeper:

"You're stupid! Your husband is stupid! Get out of here!"

She demeans Jonathan, referring to him as "the boy," never once addressing him by name. This incenses Ivy.

"I don't call Katie 'the girl.' Why do you call Jonathan 'the boy'?"

"They're not like us," Ivy commented to me once about my stepfamily.

His grandmother is not the only one enraged. Whatever anger Katie harbors is intensified by her father's tyrannical style of parenting.

Ivy watches and worries.

"She's troubled."

"I know," I say. I took her to counseling, but she didn't take it seriously.

Katie's acting-out reaches a critical point when she's involved in an incident at the mall. She's taken to the juvenile detention center, and I'm with Ivy in the kitchen when the police call.

I call Tom at work, and he waits several hours to pick her up; he wants her to learn a lesson. It's 8 p.m. when they return home.

Shortly after that incident, Ivy discovers her wedding ring missing. Convinced Katie took it, she confronts her while she plays pool in the family room with friends. I'm in the living room reading and overhear the confrontation.

"Give me my wedding ring."

"I didn't take your ring."

"I know you stole it. Give it back."

Ivy slaps her across the face, hard.

Katie bursts out crying and shouts, "You're a psycho!"

I can't believe what's happening. My mother is not aggressive.

They go their separate ways, and I find Mom in her bedroom, seething. I try to calm her with a Frank Sinatra CD. She ignores me: it's futile to try to reason with her.

I no longer can afford to do nothing about my mother's dementia. Her aggression scares me, and she has stopped talking to me. Things are out of control, and I'm frightened. The next day I make an appointment with a doctor.

A few months earlier I had attended a seminar on Alzheimer's and learned about a new medication called Exelon for those with moderate disorders. I need to learn more about this.

The ride to the doctor's office is painful. Ivy continues to display this alien personality, her face contorted and mouth curled with disdain. I'm a stranger, an enemy.

I laugh and cajole like a performer, desperate to bring her back to her "normal" self. But she stares straight ahead, her mouth twisted. The only person who understands me has now abandoned me and retreated into a place unknown. By the time I pull up to the doctor, I'm half-crazed with fear and desperation.

He interviews her and I answer for her, wanting to protect her and hold onto my denial. He ignores me. When he asks how many children she has, she responds, "Three."

"She has four."

"I guess she eliminated you," he says, laughing. I start to cry.

He gives me some samples as well as a prescription for Exelon, that new drug which, initially, upsets her stomach. Weeks pass, and I fail to see any noticeable improvement, thinking *it takes time.* When the samples are gone, my sisters and I discover its cost is astronomical and we don't fill the prescription.

Ivy's drama with Katie subsides as, unfortunately for all, it turns out her ring had been left at a friend's house when we visited months earlier. Apologies are offered, but hard feelings turn into granite.

Jonathan stays most weekends with friends. When not involved in his studies, he spends the rest of his time playing basketball for his high school team. I encourage all opportunities for him to stay away from his abusive stepfather.

This toxic environment takes its toll: Katie leaves for college in Tallahassee, and Tom's grandmother has a fatal stroke. Jonathan leaves for college, also out of town, which I encourage because I know he'll be in a safe and healthy environment.

I know I can no longer leave Ivy alone and call on an elder-care service for assistance. They send someone the next day to interview. I come home from work and, as I turn down the street, I see a striking figure in the distance, like an apparition. I feel small and pale next to her larger-than-life frame and jet-black skin. As I lower my car window, she smiles and introduces herself, a shiny gold tooth glistening in the light.

"Hi, I'm Francine."

"I'm Jennifer," I say, already relieved and comforted by her presence.

We sit in the kitchen and talk.

"She loves to play piano and take walks. But with the Alzheimer's, she gets lost and needs supervision."

"Can I meet her?"

We walk to Ivy's room, the pink-orange rays of the afternoon sun warming and softening the air.

Ivy is sitting in the straight-backed chair next to the window, her eyes closed and a blissful smile on her face as Rachmaninoff's *3rd Piano Concerto* reverberates from her silver Sony CD player.

"Hi, Mom. I want you to meet Francine. She might keep you company a couple of days a week.

"Pleased to meet you, Ivy."

"Hello," she says curtly. I had mentioned to her earlier about having a companion during the day. She didn't like the idea.

"How do you feel about spending some time with Francine, Mom?"

"Is this really necessary?" she says with pursed lips.

"I hear you love to play the piano, Ivy. I love music too, and sing in my church choir."

Ivy's expression softens.

"Would you like to play some songs on the piano, and I'll sing along?"

She hesitates, then replies,

"Do you like Gershwin?"

"Sure do!"

Their conversation continues. I arrange for Francine to come every Tuesday and Thursday for four hours, leaving her notes, requests and reminders.

"Would you take Mom to the mall? She loves to shop and needs a pair of navy Keds slip-ons, size 7-1/2."

Francine leaves me detailed, multi-page accounts of her days with Ivy, filled with singing, walks and household chores. Francine is wonderful. Her presence diffuses at least some of the negativity and tension here in the Big House.

Ivy has little to say about Francine. She doesn't really understand why she's here. But that's okay.

The Bracelet

Ivy stays with my brother Bobby and his wife for three or so weeks from time to time. Their home is less than an hour away from mine. After a recent visit, alarmed by her wandering and disorientation, they ordered an Alzheimer's bracelet for her. It arrived yesterday, and I clasped it on her right wrist without explanation. She didn't resist because she didn't really know what this was, only a silver bracelet.

It's now Sunday morning, and I'm sitting in the corner of our living room next to the stone fireplace, feet propped up on an ottoman, reading the Issues and Ideas section of *The Miami Herald*. Nature sounds abound: the delicate *cheer-cheer-cheer* of a cardinal, palm fronds flapping in the breeze and the whirring lawn mower-like sound of an ultra-light plane overhead.

I hear the soft steps of Ivy's rubber-soled shoes on our tiled floor and glance up as she steps into the living room to confront me. Raising her right arm, she pulls at the Alzheimer's bracelet with her left hand.

"I can still read, you know."

She must have noticed the inscription on the underside of the bracelet, and I see the rage seething behind her eyes.

"I know you can, Mom," I respond defensively, unprepared for this battle.

Guilt and shame seep into my chest, thick and black, like tar. My throat constricts.

"I don't need this bracelet. Take it off."

"Remember how you get lost, Mom? It'll keep you safe."

My words hang, empty and inadequate in the face of her penetrating glare.

I plead, a bad daughter who has humiliated her beloved mother by denying yet another vestige of her dignity and independence.

I have a difficult time coming to terms with my delicate mother having to wear a steel bracelet. Inscribed "Safe Return" with the Alzheimer's logo and two slanted figures joined together on the outside, its underside reads "*Memory Impaired. To help Ivy call 1-800-572-1122*," followed by her ID number.

"Take it off," her voice and gaze steely, like the bracelet. "Now!"

I eventually give in, unable to stand having her angry and upset at me. Maybe she'll be okay without it, I tell myself, though not really believing it.

The bracelet isn't easy to unclasp, and I struggle for several minutes before finally freeing her.

"There. That's better," she says, turning away, her head held high as she returns to her room. I watch her, not knowing what I feel anymore.

She's scheduled to visit my brother Bobby again in a few days. I call to tell him what happened. When he and his wife arrive to take her, I hand him the bracelet when she isn't looking. He slips it into his pocket. I hate secrets and feel as if I've betrayed her.

Maybe he'll do better, I say to myself. And he did – his son put it on her wrist, saying that this was a special gift. I breathe a sigh of relief. Yet another battle won.

Abandon Ship

I no longer recognize myself in the mirror. Somehow I allowed my hairdresser to bleach my honey-wheat blond hair. It's a cheap look, but it wasn't cheap. I don't seem to be in control anymore.

I feel like a fat, frayed shipwreck. The only time in my life I was overweight was when I was pregnant. I never had a problem before. Once calm and controlled, in charge of my life – at least most of the time – I'm on the verge of a nervous breakdown. I know this is true. "Jenna isn't herself," my sisters say.

I've been seeing a psychologist for several months now, and was told that I had anxiety. Tom came with me once, but he doesn't really believe in therapy or introspection...I think he feels threatened by it.

I loved to draw and paint as a child, but lost my confidence and didn't take art up again until my '20s. I'm painting again now after years of inactivity and a lurking self-doubt, and I share my work with my therapist in search of hidden clues to my psyche. It's a major excavation as I dig through all the muck in search of my real self. A difficult task, to be sure, but I think it's helping.

My studio/sitting room is adjacent to our bedroom. I'm reading books on spirituality and ways to overcome insurmountable obstacles: Caroline Myss, Wayne Dyer, and Sylvia Browne. I have dozens more of my favorite books, many collected during college, graduate school and beyond, stacked every which way in my built-in bookcase, like supplies in anticipation of an active hurricane season or unforeseen hardship. They comfort me.

I claim this space as my own and suspect there must be an unspoken energy field here, telling Tom to "Keep Out!"

An easel in front of the sliding-glass doors that overlook our balcony reminds me of the one my parents bought me when I was eight. They gave me a small box filled with a beginner's set of oil paints, linseed oil and a small canvas panel. Inspired by a Christmas card, I proudly recreated its sleigh-ride scene – it made me proud.

Another favorite painting was inspired by the musical *Oliver*. After seeing the film I painted a portrait of the Artful Dodger in his black top hat and coat, a white scarf draped around his shoulders with flair. I was in junior high school then, and Bobby had driven a friend and me to art class Saturday mornings on the top floor of an old firehouse station with large picture windows.

I now sit high upon a stool, my feet planted firmly on its horizontal rungs, ready to explore and expand my world, to paint my way to a new life.

Outside, from my balcony where Chris lounges in the white canvas butterfly chair while I paint, I can see my favorite gardenia bush, a tabebuia tree with its yellow blossoms and our orchid house, nestled amongst thick tropical foliage. Many birds visit, mostly blue jays, cardinals and mourning doves. Once I saw a painted bunting and a gathering of robins following their migration, both special moments.

One unwelcome visitor is a fearless, ravenous raccoon. Unfazed by humans, he eats our cats' food. I'm obsessed with this creature and want it to go away. I decide to buy a BB gun, though the only gun I ever held or owned was a water pistol. The sales clerk shows me several options, and I pick the cheapest one. Empowered in a perverse way after loading it, one pellet at a time, I stand on the upstairs balcony and aim at a tree near the orchid house. Later I place it in the top left drawer of my precious antique chest of drawers that once held Jonathan's baby clothes and remains in what is now my sacred space.

The next day when I see the raccoon climb up a tree near the kitchen, I quietly open the screen. It scurries over the roof, its toenails making a scraping sound on the shingles. Staring straight ahead with its black, beady eyes, it jumps onto the balcony and makes a beeline for the cat dish. I wait until it finishes gorging itself and watch as it dips its nose into the water dish, gulping and gurgling as the water splashes in every direction, leaving a primitive, dank smell.

As the raccoon turns around to leave, my pulse quickens as I aim right between its eyes. Shaky and unpracticed, I miss completely. Startled, it retreats. My hands shake as I shoot again and hit its backside. The pellet bounces off its greasy hide like oil from a hot frying pan.

I continue to stalk it, determined to perfect my skills. I've never encountered this predatory side of me before, and enjoy my new sport. Raccoons are clever, and it always anticipates my presence. Somehow I manage to hit it repeatedly, but not where it counts.

Weeks pass and I grow steadier. Quieter, too. I no longer wait until the raccoon finishes eating. He again approaches, and I steel my gaze and aim. No longer shaky or unskilled, I'm calm and collected and hit it right between the eyes. Bulls-eye!

Don't mess with my cat's food. It isn't yours – and don't mess with my family, Tom! I hear somewhere in the shadow of my mind.

For a moment I feel vindicated, but my triumphant moment is short-lived. Defiant and proud, the raccoon stares me down as the pellet bounces off its head like an over-inflated beach ball.

This scene entertains Tom. I'm embarrassed. What's happening to me? I'm not an aggressive person; it's not my nature. As a child I would bring home injured baby birds and nurse them back to health in the middle of the night with drops of water squeezed from an eye dropper. *I think I'm displacing my anger.*

I put the BB gun back in the drawer for good.

Painting feels more comfortable. After a decade of inactivity, I'm determined to paint again. I try not to plan ahead. It's more authentic when I allow my art to flow. My first painting looks like a Middle-Eastern woman with a large white cross around her neck, a white headdress draping her black wavy hair. She's a strong woman, beaten down by life, her eyes empty and sad...so very sad.

I'm determined to save myself. I sign up for a yoga/meditation class that meets twice a week. After a few sessions I have to quit because there is something wrong with my back.

I continue to paint a series of females in different states of being. What I see is giving me strength and clarity. These women stare at me; I feel as if they are somehow saving my life.

Don't let him beat you down. There is a way out, they seem to say.

One painting that inspires me is a nude, fluid and ethereal, in blue, green and gold. Arms outstretched, she looks is if she's moving into some other world filled with swirls, bursts of movement and energy. An unfinished figure stands next to her, *upright.* I call my painting *Transformation,* because it seems to be adopting an entirely different state of being, one free from pain and suffering. This is one of my favorite pieces and gives me hope.

I notice that I now often fly in my dreams, something that I first experienced as a child. I asked my therapist about this "out-of-body experience," and was told this was called "astral projection" and, when under extreme stress, it can occur frequently.

Flying in my dreams is the most exhilarating experience, unlike any other. My senses are heightened. The colors are golden and rosy as I fly over terrain, brushing treetops and soaring aloft, touching clouds. I'm often unaware of where I am in time, place or dimension. The terrain resembles earth, often rugged and mountainous, and sometimes I seem to be in the past.

A few months ago I was half-awake one morning and saw what appeared to be a tall Native American Indian standing outside my window with a look of deep concern. I made the mistake of asking Tom if he saw him, too, but my husband looked at me as if I were psychotic. I recognized that Indian because I had seen him in my dreams as a little girl flying over the apple orchard in our back yard in Ohio. He must be looking out for me. This too, gives me comfort.

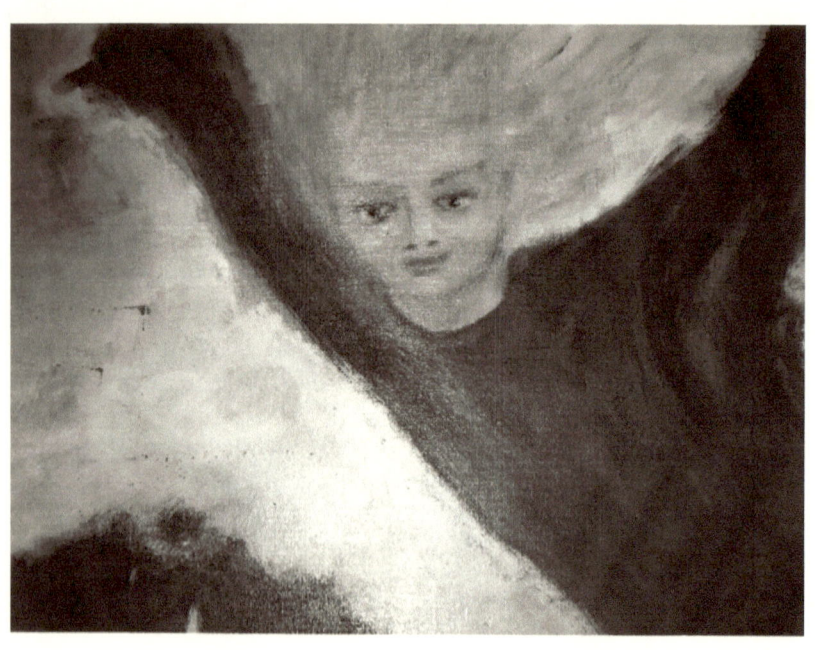

Flying Dreams

Letting Go

I can't stand living like this any longer. Tom is disengaged and distant most of the time. Our conversation is superficial, involving only day-to-day minutiae. In a way, I feel some relief. But living in limbo is making me crazy.

In addition to my emotional pain I'm in excruciating physical agony from a herniated disk pinching my sciatic nerve. Unable to stand straight, I limp around with my torso leaning to the left. Tom finds this funny, and mimics my awkward gait, pretending he's the Hunchback of Notre Dame. I'm not the only one who's the butt of his jokes; it's also open season on Ivy and Jonathan.

Last night Tom and I sat in the family room and faced our wretched reality. We both know it's not working.

"It's hard to imagine a future with someone so cruel to my son," I tell him.

"You make me sound like a louse."

I turn to him, but say nothing. The bitterness in my eyes says it all: it's over.

We continue to sitting in silence, in the same place where Ivy announced months ago that she was losing her mind.

I cry with relief and sadness, sadness for me, for my son and for my mother. Tom cries, too.

The next morning my search begins, secretly, for a new home. Weeks pass, then Tom joins in, saying little, as though in denial.

I am unable to walk more than several feet before the pain becomes intolerable and I must sit. Tom wheels me around in his grandmother's red walker as we search for a new place for me. He is dutiful like that, accustomed to overseeing the details of housing the infirmed – my mother, his grandmother. I'm now relegated to a similar lot.

Some weeks into our quest, Tom notices an ad in *The Miami Herald* for an unusual townhouse near downtown Miami on a wooded lot. I love the idea of living in the city after nine years in comparative isolation. With its abundance of trees, this should be an easy transition. The notion of becoming a part of a community again is appealing.

We arrange to meet the realtor on a Sunday morning. There's 'round-the-clock security and, after passing through the guarded gate, we park in the garage beneath the compound. The owner invites us in. His two-story townhome is open and airy with floor-to-ceiling windows that line the rear of its ground level, much like those in the living room of the Big House. The view is similar, too: mature trees, palms, bromeliads and an abundance of tropical foliage. The owner recently renovated his unit with impeccable taste and is justifiably proud.

At the end of our tour, I know this is right for me. It looks like an artist's studio and, with neighbors, safe. I'll have a place to garden and, hopefully, a home where I can not only survive, but thrive.

Facing Reality

The time has come for me to make a decision about Ivy's care. Her needs are acute, and I can no longer care for her. My strength is compromised; I can barely walk.

I make phone calls, talk to co-workers, scour the yellow pages and surf the Internet. I drive around the city, limping my way through tours of assorted facilities. Many have waiting lists, so my options are limited. My final visit is to a facility near the Big House. A friend of a friend's mother loves it there. It's relatively small, self-contained and clean, with a feng shui design to foster harmony. A skylight in its foyer radiates light and airiness. An administrator shares that her grandmother had Alzheimer's; she understands. While touring the main wing, I must sit often due to the piercing pain on my left side. The administrator has also suffered from sciatica and understands.

The cost is affordable, so I call my siblings to tell them about this facility. They view its website and offer no alternatives. With trepidation, we all agree. The decision has been made.

Another painful decision concerns my back. Months have passed, and my doctor offers little support or guidance.

Walking is difficult without a walker or crutches. I moan at night; I cry.

"Will you stop crying? I can't sleep," Tom complains.

His lack of compassion intensifies my pain. I ask the doctors for painkillers, but am denied, as surgery is recommended. After a second opinion confirming surgery is needed, an operation is scheduled...finally.

I tell Jonathan who is away at college. Knowing Tom will give me no comfort in this ordeal, I ask one of my sisters to travel from Ohio for help. Annie takes leave of her employer and arrives within days. The cavalry is here, thank God.

Annie drives me to the hospital early November 18 for surgery. I limp and stagger down the corridor to pre-op, my sister at my side.

"Can you make it, Jenna?" she asks with concern.

I lean against the wall, feeling faint, when a nurse offers me a wheelchair.

"Yes, please. I can't walk anymore."

Time passes quickly. I'm not afraid. I just want the pain to go away.

When I awaken from surgery, my mouth is parched, and I panic. "I can't breathe! Help me!"

I'm given chips of ice, and then wheeled into a room where the next 24 hours are nothing less than a nightmare.

Every nerve ending at the site of the incision is on fire. The more I struggle against the pain, the more it intensifies. The nurses ask that I measure it from one to ten, but my pain far surpasses ten.

"Annie, please tell them it's more than a ten. Please."

"I'll tell them again. But they say you have to wait another four hours for morphine," she says helplessly.

"Please. Beg them."

It's nightfall now, and I'm in a place I pray I'll never see again. How can I describe my pain? Searing, piercing, debilitating, agonizing, stabbing, burning, unbearable, incapacitating – I know them all. I have an intimate relationship with pain and suffering.

The surgeon arrives the next morning, chipper and sporting a red bowtie, an eccentric, professor-type.

Informed by the nurses I was a difficult patient, he looks at me with a disappointed expression. I'm guilty – I shouldn't have begged for more morphine.

"I hear you had a difficult night." He studies me intently. I just stare at him, afraid to move.

"You don't really want to stay here another night, do you?"

He makes it sound so simple. I'm stunned.

"I'm in a lot of pain."

"I need you to try to walk."

He can't be serious. I don't feel anything but a knife in my back. Do my legs still work?

"I can't walk. Really."

I don't know why, but I like this man and trust him. "Here, let me help you sit up. Let's try to stand up now. I'll hold you."

"No, I can't. Really, I can't." I wince as the pain radiates down my leg.

But somehow I stand, walk and three hours later am discharged.

Annie drives me home where I soon discover the pain eases if I keep moving. I shuffle gingerly around the house, telling myself, "Don't stop, Jennifer, don't stop. Life will get better."

The Center

Ivy is scheduled to move to the assisted living center the day after Thanksgiving.

"We're both moving uptown, Mom. I'm moving to a townhouse, and you're moving to a place where you'll be well cared for."

I'm trying to stay upbeat and convincing, but I know I've betrayed her.

"Why can't I go with *you*?"

My argument is empty. She doesn't understand.

My sisters and I pack her clothes, family photos and whatever else we think she would choose if she were in her right mind.

I grab the yellow lunchbox containing her many medications, its exterior a collage of photos, musical symbols and colorful mementos in sharp contrast with its life-saving contents. There are ten of us, so we take two cars to what we believe will be our mother's final home. We pass a small coral rock house flanked by avocado and orange groves, and a weathered Latino sporting a straw hat, sitting on a lawn chair next to a mound of papayas in the back of his pick-up truck. When we reach our destination, the staff is waiting for us, but mom still doesn't understand what is happening.

"Hi Ivy," the blond administrator beams and gives her a hug. Her name is Mari, and she greets our assembled clan: "Are you Cuban?"

No one can muster up any laughter, as we walk through the double-glass doors into an atrium with a parquet-wood floor. Overhead is a skylight, and late afternoon rays filter down on us, while a portrait of the mother of the founder of this facility, who also suffered from Alzheimer's, is prominently positioned on the wall above a honey-colored organ. The atmosphere is bright, and everyone is smiling.

Mari escorts all ten of us to the end of the hallway, past the nurses' station.

"Here's your room, Ivy, and this is Rose who will be your roommate."

Mom's eyes dart back and forth. Her breathing accelerates.

"I don't want to be here. I want to go home."

"Look at this pretty room, Mom. You have a beautiful view of the grounds."

A labyrinth of shrubbery dotted with white blossoms winds around an otherwise empty back lot. Cement benches adorned with pastel motifs are strategically placed at either end.

Rose, who looks to be in her late '70s or early '80s, sits scowling in the chair next to the window. Neatly dressed, she appears somewhat reserved and not particularly welcoming. We're told she was once a math teacher.

"She isn't going to cause problems, is she?" Rose says, her eyes glaring, ready for battle. "Maybe she needs to be in the locked wing."

She's accustomed to her privacy, I suspect, and would rather be alone.

"Now Rose, don't be rude," Mari says, also agitated.

"I'm just saying she might be better off in the locked wing." Rose speaks with the authority of someone used to being in charge.

We unpack Ivy's belongings and carefully set the family photos on a shelf alongside her bed. I had made a special flower arrangement of yellow, pink and orange silk flowers in a ceramic vase decorated with purple petunias that I gave her long ago, and set this on her nightstand.

"I don't want to be here. This isn't my home."

"Grandma, you're moving uptown now," says my nephew. "It's a nice place. Give it a try."

Peggy hands the lunchbox containing medication and critical documents to Mari. Jonathan and his cousins leave the room, electing not to witness the increasingly desperate scene.

The conversation continues to go round and round, like a slowly moving carousel. I want to get off – but can't.

Mom won't be persuaded. Guilt is crashing down on me like glass shards. I sit on the bed, weary and pained. It would be *so* much easier if she went along, I say to myself.

The carousel continues its torturous spin.

"I'm not going to stay here a minute longer."

"Come on, Mom. It's not so bad."

Rose continues to badger us like a relentless beaver until Ivy, thankfully, is assigned to another room.

Three hours elapse, with Mari staying past her usual departure time.

"Keep an eye on Ivy tonight," she warns her replacement, fingers pointing to her eyes for emphasis. Although I have no recollection of our eventually leaving, I clearly recall abandoning my mother.

The phone rings the next morning.

"Your mother didn't have a good night. She kept trying to leave. She was extremely agitated and was walking around naked."

Ivy hates her new home. I visit her every single day and take her outside, convincing myself she'll adapt. Less than a week later, I get another call.

"We think your mother needs to be moved to the Alzheimer's wing."

I've seen this wing and can't imagine my mother living there. I call my siblings. We're backed into a corner. What are our options?

They lock my mother away.

I'm still recuperating from back surgery and unable to return to work, but manage to drive to the Center. With both dread and despair, I rescue her for a few hours a day without fail. I push the button to open the locked doors, trying to ease our pain and my guilt. Patients are lined up on either side of the corridor, some deep in conversation with themselves or the person next to them, word salads tossed every which way. Some are screaming, others babbling and drooling with empty eyes and squelched spirits, discarded beings like the stuffed animals and dolls that rest on their laps, substitutes for lost loved ones. At its end are a nurses' station and a TV suspended from the ceiling. Residents hover here, some shuffling papers, others sleeping upright. How can my mother be in a place like this? Something is terribly wrong.

A man holding onto his walker repeatedly screams,

"Gimme five! Gimme five! Gimme five!"

Most speak Spanish; many scream. The aides are smiling, but I don't think they're particularly happy. Neither Ivy nor I fit in here.

Residents are locked out of their rooms during the day so their whereabouts might be monitored. Evie, Ivy's new roommate, is relatively young, perhaps in her '60s. Always smiling, she nods her head in agreement to everything, her shoulder-length blond hair pulled back with a barrette. She's always caring for a stuffed animal that she caresses protectively on her lap.

"Hi, Evie."

"Hello, dear. God bless you."

Her words soften the harshness.

As I walk down the corridor, the alarm sounds. Ivy approaches me, shrugging her shoulders as she covers her ears to block the deafening noise. She loves to take walks and tried to leave through the back door.

She sees me, and her face lights up.

"Doll! You saved me!"

Our eyes meet. She smiles, but her expression hints at the internal struggle in her brain.

We hold each other tight. I clasp her hand while punching in the security code. We push open the door open and emerge onto the parquet-wood floor to be greeted by the sparkling sun's golden rays. Ivy sighs with relief.

"Oh! This is beautiful!"

We walk hand-in-hand to the registration desk to sign out. Tiny parakeets chirp and flutter all about the cage near the window. They want to escape, too.

Residents and family members sit in floral upholstered chairs flanking the windows. I make a mental note of the two contrasting worlds only feet apart – the Alzheimer's wing, a skeleton in the closet I'm not yet able to come to terms with.

Ivy and I blink to adjust our eyes as we come out into the welcome sunlight, our moods immediately uplifted.

Moving Day

Four weeks have passed since my back surgery, twenty days since Ivy's move to the Center. It's the first day of my new life.

I know that nothing will ever be the same again. The pain from my surgery is healing, but I realize the pain from years of emotional and verbal abuse will take far longer to heal. The left side of my leg and foot are numb from sciatic nerve damage. I wonder if this is a physical manifestation of the emotional numbness that seemed to safeguard me from my husband's rage, his lengthy irrational silences, his sarcasm and put-downs, abuses and vulgarity. I know things will never be the same again, but when I *am* able to feel again, I know it will be good.

I've packed my possessions. Boxes and furniture are tagged. The movers are due this morning.

The phone rings at 5 a.m., and my heart jumps. I've been awake for hours.

"Hello?"

"Jennifer?"

"Yes, who's this?"

"This is Mari from the Center. Your mother is okay, but she had to be taken to the hospital. She was having trouble breathing."

In addition to Alzheimer's, Ivy suffers from chronic obstructive pulmonary lung disease and emphysema. She's also asthmatic.

"Is she all right?" *Please let her be okay...please*, I say to myself.

"She's going to be all right. The ambulance took her to Baptist Hospital a few minutes ago."

"I'll be there shortly."

I hang up; dress in ten seconds and race to the hospital in the dark.

Ivy is in a cubicle in the emergency room, hooked up to oxygen. Her eyes are closed. We hold hands.

Instructed to sit in the waiting room, I find a seat facing the window. Already exhausted, I close my eyes and try to organize the disordered thoughts bouncing around in my head. I need to get through this day in one piece, I tell myself. An industrial clock overhead reads 7:15 a.m. I'm reminded of the old clock in my elementary school and sigh – how carefree those days those were!

Outside a grimy window, the splendor of the rising sun calms my nerves. Inside, the routine is familiar. I sat in this same waiting room with Jonathan 11 years ago. He'd cracked his skull open to the bone during soccer practice. His coach, who spoke only broken English, called to tell me he was injured, providing neither details nor comfort. I sped to the soccer field, fearing the worst. His teammates ran over to my car, escorting me to the school office as we followed a trail of my son's blood. The paramedics were at his side, bandages wrapped about his head like a turban. I had taken him to this same emergency room.

I don't remember how many stitches he was given, but what I do recall is the doctor's tales of the aftermath of Hurricane Andrew. He told us about a boy my son's age that hid in a closet with his dog. The dog panicked, biting the boy's head, also to the bone. But he survived, like Jonathan, only another battle scar to be borne with pride.

Ivy is stable and in good hands, so I leave the hospital at 9 a.m. The movers are already at the house. Their van is too big for our winding driveway, so they park on the street and use Tom's small truck to transport my possessions to their van.

Two hours later they finish. My car is also loaded, so I fasten my seatbelt and move slowly down the driveway. As its stones crackle under the tires, I begin to relax, feeling the burden of my former life being lifted ever so slowly. Overhead the birds soar freely, while tree snails crawl up the trees as nature thrives in all its glory. I gaze in my rearview mirror to see Cleo and Patch follow me to the end of the driveway, the only inhabitants there to say goodbye. In their eyes I imagine a kindred yearning to escape too, to leave this beautiful, horrible place. I apologize silently to them and inch past the cedar gate, turning north...toward a new beginning.

The Ladies Lunch

Ivy and I are both trying to adjust to her new home. Saturday, without fail, is our day to lunch. I live on the other side of Miami, so this has become a half-day excursion. The first Saturday after I settled in, I brought her to see my new place and made lunch for the two of us.

"Jenna, it's elegant!"

I want her to come upstairs and see my paintings, but she fears my spiral staircase. It confuses her.

"I'll help you, Mom. Don't be afraid."

I walk behind and hold her as we circle upward, step by step, then hold her hand as we walk into the bedroom.

"This is my latest painting, Mom. What do you think?"

"I love it."

Ivy always encouraged me as an artist. In elementary school I used to draw on the cardboard inserts from her Hanes hosiery packages. She saved all my sketches in a purple shoebox, and I still have these. One in particular is of me at the age of eight or so, in a sailor outfit, holding a bouquet of flowers behind my back as I stand in front of her, my long blond hair pulled back with a barrette. She leans forward, smiling, an apron tied around her waist and her hands folded, waiting in anticipation for her surprise. It sits on my desk.

Soon after my move, I hire a landscaper to install a small pond and waterfall in my patio. Ivy and I sit outside and eat lunch. We talk and laugh. Birds and squirrels are busy in the surrounding treetops, while a lizard darts along the stucco wall. We listen as the waterfall gurgles over the rocks, the city sounds in the background softened by the sounds of nature. Ivy and I celebrate my new home, my new life.

Our Saturdays together become a ritual, and we almost always eat at one of several restaurants close to the Center where she lives. I notice a change in her attire as the months pass, as her clothing becomes part a communal supply.

So I'm never certain what to expect when I visit her.

She has gone through what could be described as a "flapper" stage with short, flippy skirts, cardigan sweaters and white ankle socks that complement her refreshing, free-spirited demeanor. Even the soft wavy curls of her hair match her now-girlish ways. No longer is Ivy "a proper woman" who represses unpleasant feelings and preserves the amenities; she's newly transformed, liberated and uncensored.

During a recent stroll amid the labyrinth out back she exclaimed, "This is beautiful...like sex!" I gasp, embarrassed but happy for her freedom from repression.

I too am slowly transforming my life, finding my way back. No longer on high alert, I notice and appreciate "the little gifts of life" I've been missing for so long: the kindness of neighbors and convenience of city life, new friends, classes at the downtown college campus. Sleeping peacefully is also a newly discovered gift, as my back is becoming stronger.

I've also come to expect the unexpected when Ivy and I are together.

"Jenna, when did you sail into town?"

"I just arrived today. Isn't that great?"

"Are we having a wild anticipation?"

"We are!"

"Let's do something Oriental."

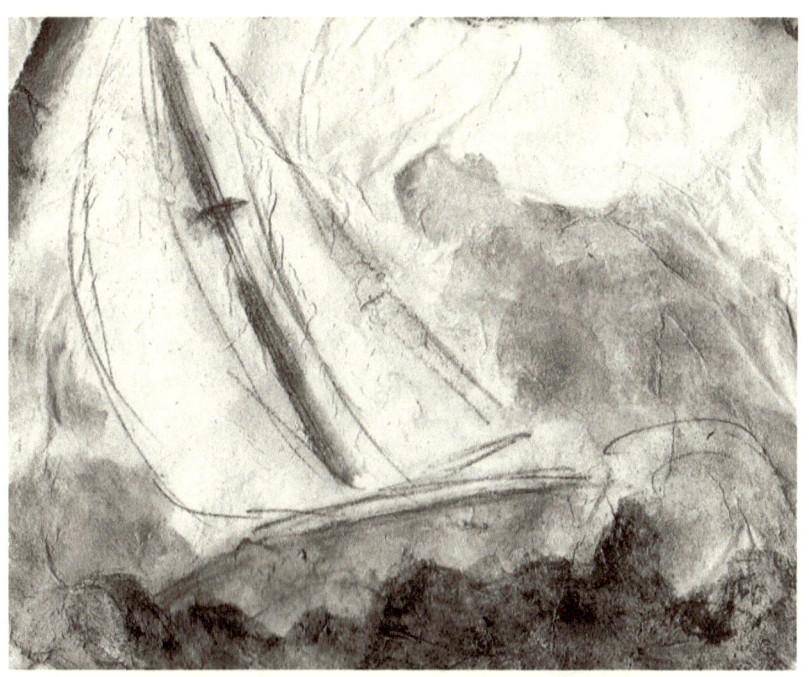

Jenna, when did you sail into town?

"I thought we'd do something breezy...like Bahama Breeze."

"Don't tell anyone."

"Never."

Bahama Breeze is one of our favorite restaurants. We love its tropical-colored walls and plates. It's casual and colorful, evoking cherished memories. Their bold palette matches the walls in my first home – ultramarine blue, celadon green and terra cotta orange. Ivy helped me choose those colors. Like my new townhouse, this looked like an artist's studio.

My father was alive then. He and Ivy spent months with Jonathan and me to escape the cold, dreary winters up north. After decorating the interior of my first home, Ivy and I would garden, hoisting pavers, hauling trees and dragging 100-pound bags of topsoil around. I have fond memories of my mother standing alongside its entrance, arms up, feet wide like a warrior, perfecting the placement of a traveler's palm we were planting. We were pioneer women driven by our boundless imagination and energy. We could do it all.

Jonathan was young, and my parents adored him, my father calling him, "my little man." We all took long walks, gazed at the sunsets from our balcony and, unfailingly, looked after one another.

Ivy and I sit in a booth by the window at Bahama Breeze, pretending we're on a Caribbean holiday. Small green, yellow, coral and blue plates brighten the table. One of her favorite dishes is black bean soup, always with a dollop of sour cream on top. She loves soup – and the word *dollop*. I must order for her now; menus no longer make sense. I order a quesadilla. Both our entrees are accompanied by glasses of chardonnay.

We lift our glasses.

"Cheers!"

"Such riches! I love my life! But Doll, you need to teach me to talk again. What is it that you think with? Ears? Cats?"

"You think with your mind, Mom. Don't worry; I understand you."

She flirts with the waiter, a clean-cut Latino in his '20s. When he leaves with our order, she comments in a sultry tone, "I'd like to have more of that."

"Mom!"

We indulge ourselves with a layered chocolate almond dessert topped with whipped cream, savoring every bite. This inspires Ivy, and she breaks into poetry for the first time in months, beginning with *The Highwayman.* I fill in the blanks, and we end with *Thanatopsis.*

"Jenna! We're one!"

"We are. Isn't that beautiful?"

I pay the check and hold her hand as we walk to the car. Our hearts soar. As we approach the Center, Ivy smiles at me and asks, "Doll, have you been to the moon?"

"No. Would you like to go?"

"I'd love to!"

She smiles and nods; her eyes glisten. *We're flying to the moon!* I wonder if she, like me, flies at night. In our world anything is possible.

We enter the locked wing, and I walk her to an empty chair along the wall. We hug and kiss goodbye. She places her hands over her ears and closes her eyes, smiling.

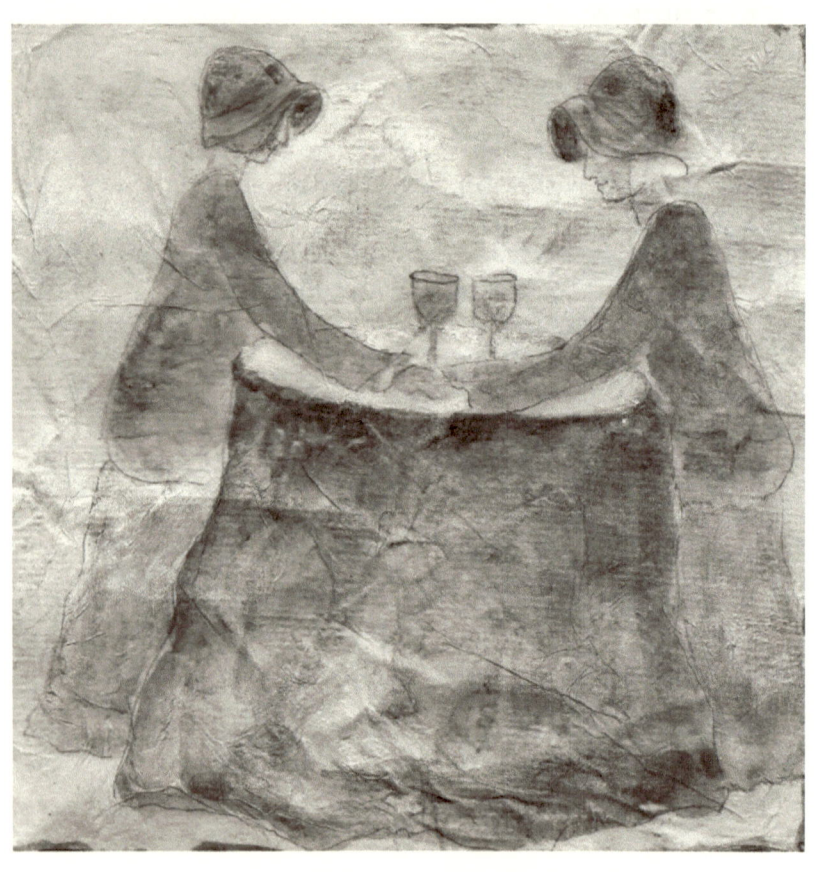

The Ladies Lunch

Falling

A year has passed since my mother moved into the Alzheimer's wing, and she continues to fall. Often.

I'm at work when the phone rings. I pick it up on the first ring, ever on high alert.

"Jennifer?"

"Yes."

"This is Mari from the Center. It's not an emergency, but your mother fell and is at the emergency room."

I've somehow come to appreciate the standard line, "It's not an emergency." This makes the bad news that always follows more bearable.

The all-too-familiar wave of anxiety washes through my body. Shaking hands and a dry mouth follow.

"Is she okay?"

"She's going to be all right, but she cut her lip."

I've forgotten how many times she has fallen, but what I can't forget are my panic and tears, fleeing work at a moment's notice, not knowing for certain what I'll find upon arrival at the emergency room.

A few months ago, Ivy's lip was cut, her right hand and arm so bruised and swollen that the Alzheimer's bracelet was embedded in her skin, cutting off her circulation. I alerted a nurse and they began to search for a tool that would cut through steel. A half-hour later an aide, young, heavy-set with kind eyes, arrived carrying what looked like pliers.

"See? It's on her right arm. Her circulation is getting cut off."

"Let me take a look."

The aide lifted Ivy's arm and realized it was going to be a challenge not to cut her tissue-paper-like skin, now swollen around the bracelet. He worked at it for ten minutes, but to no avail.

"I don't think these will work. Let me see what else I can find."

The nurse checks Ivy's arm again and talks to the young man. He walks away and soon returns with a smaller tool.

"Let's try this."

She pushes some gauze under the clasp and together they try to free her. I see he's determined; I'm grateful.

Twenty minutes pass until he finally cuts her loose.

"Got it!" he says.

"Thank God! Thank you so much."

He hands me the severed bracelet, and I start to breathe freely again.

The nurse checks her wrist and gently massages it.

"She'll be fine."

I'm brought back to the present as I pull into the hospital grounds. I find Ivy lying on a cot in the hallway, the shape of my mother's upper lip is permanently altered from all of her many lacerations. I'm amazed and thankful she hasn't broken any bones.

The emergency aide from the ambulance is by her side, required to look after her until an authorized person arrives. Ivy's mouth is the size of a tennis ball.

"Mom!"

She smiles with her twisted mouth, and her eyes sparkle in that loving and familiar way.

"Jenna! You saved me!" This is Ivy's standard response to such situations, and her elation eases my anxiety.

"You sure know how to have a good time, Mom," I tease.

The paramedic asks, "Are you Ivy's daughter?"

"Yes."

"You need to sign here."

As I sign the paper, a handsome young doctor with dark eyes walks up, his manner confident and easy-going.

"Are you Ivy?" he says.

"Yes, she is."

I have to stop this habit. Let *her* answer, I tell myself.

He smiles at me, directing his attention only to my mother.

"Hello, Ivy."

She smiles her crooked smile, looking him up and down, studying every inch of his physique. In a deep, sultry voice, she responds, "Well, hello there."

She's now a 90-year-old seductress with a tennis-ball mouth ready to seduce a young doctor.

He laughs and asks her several questions, making a point of talking only to her. I try to keep quiet.

She continues her flirtations, answering as best she can.

The comedy is short-lived. He tells us that a plastic surgeon is on his way and will sew her mouth up "like new." Again.

Fifteen minutes elapse, and the surgeon, tanned and looking as if he just stepped off a tennis court, greets us.

"What happened, Ivy? You fell again?"

She nods.

They wheel her into the room and close the curtain. "Please be careful. She's fragile."

I don't know what I'm saying. Of course they know she's fragile.

"I'll be right out here, Mom. You'll be okay." I hate this.

I wait in the hall with Mari who has come from the Center to make certain the situation is well in hand. I hear my mother scream, and my stomach lurches.

"I came here for a good time!" she wails.

My head feels like a helium balloon, so I sit down. Tears that have been bottled up burst forth, and a nurse's aide steps from behind the curtain to check on me.

"Are you all right? Would you like a glass of water?"

"I'll be okay." I force the words out between spastic breaths.

Mari rubs my back and tries to console me.

"Your mom will be fine. I know how hard this is."

It's over in a matter of minutes. Discharge papers are signed and instructions spelled out. It's almost 9 p.m. now, so I decide to take Mom home in my car rather than request an ambulance. I want her next to me as long as possible. Several staff members greet her with open arms, and I escort her into the Alzheimer's wing where her dinner waits. I hug and kiss her goodbye, then drive home laughing with tears streaming down my face.

The Glow

The phone rings and I learn my mother is once again in the hospital. This time it's not due to a fall; it's a breathing problem. I leave work and rush to the hospital, an all-too-familiar routine, and park in the same place on the fourth floor of the garage, close to the elevator. Later, at night, I won't have to worry so much about getting to my car safely.

I approach the registration desk and am told Ivy's room is on the third floor. Fear announces itself in my shallow breath, parched mouth and pounding heart. I walk past the gift shop, the fluorescent lights illuminating assorted knick-knacks, helium-filled balloons and flowers, and approach the elevator. I never quite know what to expect when I walk into her room, but am thankful I won't see a lip disfigured due to a fall. No plastic surgeon to call. Breathing difficulties mean tubes in her nose and an IV in her hand.

My mother greets me with a weak but peaceful smile. I pull the red vinyl armchair forward from the corner of the room and sit beside her bed to hold her hand. I watch her chest rise and fall, protruding clavicles accentuating the flow of every breath.

"Jenna, what am I supposed to be doing?"

"Just what you're doing, Mom, resting. They sent you here to fix your breathing, so don't worry."

The hospital is under renovation and still in some disrepair. The pink-and-yellow floral wallpaper in her room is faded and peeling at the corners. Once cheerful and light, it now recedes into the wall, resigned to its demise. The room has a view, but one that's far from pleasant; it addresses an adjacent balcony with scaffolding lined with cans and assorted tools.

I feel a chill and take some extra white cotton blankets from an unattended cart, doubling these for extra warmth, then spread them over my mother. We continue to hold hands in silence.

A large Jamaican woman comes in to clean the floor and says hello.

I love the cadence of her language – it sounds like a lullaby. I return her greeting and watch to make certain she sweeps up the bandage wrapper and pill cups that were dropped on the floor. Ivy was always fastidious and would most certainly be bothered by such a mess. The cleaning lady pulls out a slopping rag doll of a mop and moves it rhythmically around the room. She and the rag doll mop evoke happy childhood memories, my sisters and I playing with abandon while Maude, our cleaning lady, moves with authority in the same deliberate way, in and out and all around us. We dare not get in her way for fear of her wrath. The Jamaican woman thrusts her mop under my chair, and I lift my feet obediently. The industrial smell of the cleaner is reassuring. Someone is in control.

I continue my reverie with images of the Ohio countryside, surrounded by family, neighbors and friends. Our playground is verdant and expansive, fueling my imagination. I imagine the scent of wet cut grass after a summer thunderstorm that explodes before my eyes outside the tall picture windows on opposite sides of our living room. I love that smell and Mother Nature's light show. At dusk, lightning bugs flash on and off like miniature fireworks. My sisters and I gently embrace them with cupped hands and place them in an empty, newly-washed Hellmann's mayonnaise jar. We poke holes through the metal screw top lid so they can breathe. The show continues in the blackness of our bedrooms before we go to sleep. We'll set them free the next morning.

Our front yard is bordered on one side by a ravine lined with maples, pin oaks, a buckeye tree and native shrubs. A shallow creek winds its way over and around stones of all shapes and sizes. We negotiate a path of river rocks to the other side, at times slipping and sloshing through the water as it seeps through our well-worn white Keds and cotton bobby socks. I love the mud and messiness of childhood.

"Mom, I got a wet foot!" I shout out as the screened door slams behind me in our breezeway "mud room."

Our driveway, covered with a thin layer of white gravel, stretches from the road past our cousins' house to the garage. One of our blue-green Frasier fir Christmas trees towers on the left. Nestled in the corner is our playhouse, made from leftover planks of wood from the house and painted green. One summer Peggy and I dismantled the floor in hopes of transforming it into a barn for the pony we never got. A red metal swing set and teeter-totter are placed near a pear tree planted by my uncle. This is a perfect setting for play: softball, tag, kickball, croquet and our all-time favorite, kick-the-can.

"Ally Ally in free!" we yell with exuberance.

A dinner bell, heavy and rusted that hangs to the left of our cousins' kitchen door, clangs like clockwork at 6 p.m. during the long summer months as our aunt calls out in a melodic, alto voice,

"Dinner!"

We're loved, unconditionally. I feel safe – and free.

My mother's breathing problems frighten me far more than her falls. I start to think about our many trips to the hospital during the past 20 years, some in my car and some in an ambulance, as she was choking and gasping for breath. I've lost count of the number of times she's been at death's door with a tube down her throat, unable to breathe on her own.

It's winter and we're at the Big House. I hear a pounding sound coming from her room around 4 a.m. She's on the floor, banging the door against the wall to get my attention, her face practically blue. Terrified and shaking, I call 911. I sit next to her and cradle her in my arms until the paramedics arrive. She spends several days in intensive care. I don't leave her side. We communicate by writing. Her hand trembles, but she writes legibly, "Am I dying?"

Another evening her breathing is somewhat labored. I make certain that she takes her medicine and inhalers, then reluctantly go to bed. Work was stressful, and I'm so tired. I try to convince myself Ivy will be all right.

Three hours later she knocks on my door, breathless, mouthing, "I can't breathe." I call 911 and ride in the ambulance with her to the hospital. The next morning I sit in the hospital lounge, sobbing on the phone to my sister Peggy, "I shouldn't have gone to bed! Why did I go to bed?!"

My mother spends several days in the ICU with a tube down her throat. This is one hospital stay when the morphine causes hallucinations. I'm shocked when the nurses inform me the night before my mother told them a man in a trench coat had stolen her jewelry. They can't be talking about my mother. She wouldn't make up a story like that; they must be confused.

I sit here now wondering how many more times she will skirt death. She doesn't have a tube down her throat, but she looks so frail and defeated. I'm frightened and feel a surge of overwhelming sadness. Tears begin to cascade down my face, but I don't want my mother to know I'm crying so I continue to smile. For whatever reason, I feel as if this might be the end...the last few moments of her life. We're the only two people in the world. We gaze lovingly at each other. She smiles at me and begins to nod her head again and again, staring into my eyes. Yes, yes, she says without speaking. Yes. I hold onto her tightly.

Then something remarkable occurs: a soft, golden glow surrounds her and fills the room. Her luminous, light-blue eyes radiate a profound eternal love. She continues to regard me intently, nodding knowingly. Yes, yes, yes. Her gaze into my eyes is uninterrupted. We aren't in a dismal hospital room any longer. Time and place are suspended. It feels like we're in Heaven, our souls connected. They always have been. I continue to cry, my head on her chest, my hands grasping her shoulders.

I don't know how much time elapsed when the nurse returns.

"How's Ivy?"

I'm disoriented and don't respond.

She checks her vital signs.

"How is she? Is she going to be all right?"

"Don't worry. She'll be fine. The doctor makes his rounds in about an hour."

After the nurse leaves, I rest my head on my mother's lap and close my eyes.

Homecoming

The day before Hurricane Wilma is due here in South Florida, an administrator from the facility calls to inform me that Ivy's breathing was labored, so she was admitted to the hospital. I've already made my hurricane preparations, ensuring that I have on hand bottled water, canned goods, batteries, a full tank of gas in my car, plants secured under the balcony, and shutters in working order. Then I call my friend Elaine in Boca Raton, affirming that our homes are open to each other, depending upon which way the wind blows.

My mother has fallen too many times and her respiratory problems are not managed properly, so I'm relieved to learn she'll be safe in the hospital during the hurricane. Last year I was shocked to learn the Center had no back-up generator and its residents were without power for several days, confined to a dark, humid and stifling facility with flood waters lurking at its doorstep.

A week ago Peggy and I broached the subject of transferring Mom to a home in Ohio. There's one room available in its Alzheimer's wing, and she would have more professional care.

With my full tank of gas, critical for evacuation, I head to the hospital in South Dade, 18 miles from my home. As I exit the elevator, I see her lying on a bed at the end of the hallway, small, vulnerable and visibly cold, without blankets.

"Why is my mother not covered? Can't you see she's shivering?"

"She just arrived," the nurse explains, giving me several blankets so I can cover her. Ivy smiles lovingly at me as I rub her to provide additional warmth.

The hospital is abuzz with hurricane talk – anxiety and apprehension resound from its walls. Hurricane Wilma is due to make landfall tomorrow morning, its menacing red/orange mass depicted on TV, as hovering offshore. A chunky, blonde Anglo nurse wearing a pink sweater enters the room. She checks my mother's vital signs and oxygen equipment. Everything is stable.

"Are these windows hurricane-proof?" I ask.

She smiles and nods.

"The hospital was destroyed during Hurricane Andrew, then completely renovated. It's now state-of-the-art, with a back-up generator in case power goes out. We're safe."

"Are you here all night?"

"Sure am," she says unfazed. "I left my husband and kids to fend for themselves."

I can hardly contain my relief. I want her to look after my mother when Wilma arrives ashore.

Ivy is stable and in good hands, so I leave the hospital that evening to find that north-bound traffic on U.S.1 is gridlocked due to the mandatory evacuation order in the Florida Keys. I turn right from the parking lot and take the turnpike, the additional miles eating up my emergency gas reserve.

Once home, I'm thankful my son is here with me.

We watch the 'round-the-clock hysteria on TV, then close and lock the hurricanes shutters before taking our respective flashlights to our rooms.

"'Night, Jonathan."

"'Night, Mom."

Beside my bed is the small battery-operated TV, my security blanket during hurricanes. I'm reminded of Hurricane Andrew in August 1992, my first. Jonathan and I, living alone in our townhouse, had decided to stay with Tom and his children at their house a few miles to the south.

This tiny TV is a lifeline. Bryan Norcross, the CBS meteorologist, speaks with the authority of a parent in charge, calmly reassuring countless residents calling the studio, frozen with terror, crouched in closets, bathtubs, huddled under mattresses as their homes explode around them with the force of the Category-5 hurricane. Jonathan and Tom's daughter Katie, both nine years old at the time, and I stare through a small opening in the plywood covering the rear window to witness a Royal Poinciana tree fly horizontally across the yard like a child's toy. We hear the gravel from atop our roof, propelled like bullets, shatter the windows of his parked car.

We're being assaulted by a force I've never experienced. The walls and roof of this little house feel like tissue paper – it seems only a matter of time before we succumb to such power. We crouch in the hallway, and I think I'm going to die. As the violence outside intensifies, my terror turns into a full-blown anxiety attack, and I'm unable to speak or move for what seems likes hours. Jonathan, alarmed, calls out, "Tom, there's something wrong with my mom."

Tom stares at me blankly, saying nothing. When water streams through the ceiling light, he and his son place electronic equipment and small items onto the sofa before proceeding to their respective bedrooms, leaving Jonathan, Katie and me crouched on the floor in the hallway.

We survive Hurricane Andrew without injury, though the roof is severely damaged and the house is flooded with water. The surrounding terrain is transformed into an alien landscape. Helicopters hover over the city, while armed National Guardsmen are stationed in key posts to control the resultant chaos. It takes months for normalcy to return to Miami and its environs.

This is my point of reference with all hurricanes.

As Wilma approaches, I lie awake in the blackness of my bedroom, listening to increasingly eerie sounds outside the window that gradually reach a crescendo around 6:30 a.m. It's a strange symphony: wailing winds, the steady *pow-pow-pow* of debris thrust against shuttered windows and walls, and the explosion of glass and generators. I stare at the flashing numbers on my clock radio and hear little beeps from appliances as the power goes out and, with it, our creature comforts. A heavy stillness settles over us like a wet wool blanket.

The wind bursts gradually lose some of their fury, sufficiently for Jonathan and me to safely emerge and assess the damage. As we open the shutters, we hear the same *clap-clap-clap* of metal on metal as neighbors also emerge, pushing and pulling panels on rusty rails. Shards of glass from an overhead skylight pierce my contained and carefully tended garden, one bulky remnant afloat in my pond. The dracaena I recently planted is sprawled across the water, its roots ripped and exposed. Outside the wrought-iron gate, century-old native trees stand stoically, but Mother Nature has pruned them with unbridled brutality. The damage to our natural city center hammock is widespread, but mostly cosmetic. Like the native trees, we survive relatively unscathed. Jonathan and I return to our patio and systematically begin the clean-up process.

I call the hospital, always thankful for my landline, purposely bought because of hurricanes and power outages. The generator power is up and running and Ivy is stable. For this too, I am thankful.

I don't visit the hospital that day. The public is discouraged from travel, due to debris, downed power lines and mangled traffic lights. The streets are dangerous. Jonathan is preparing for law school and has a temporary job as a server at a local restaurant whose owner calls to see if he can come there to help clean up so they can reopen quickly. It's about a 20-minute walk from our townhouse.

There's some speculation that Wilma may have spawned the tornadoes that tore through Miami's Financial District, a prestigious area where this restaurant is located. Windows have blown out, and broken glass panes sprinkle the streets like crushed ice. Towering skyscrapers, once gleaming in tropical splendor, now stand imperfect and exposed, holes agape like empty eye sockets, their facades scarred and pocked. Police tape blocks pedestrians from sidewalks to shelter them from falling glass. Water gushes from a burst line.

The restaurant opens in a few days. The great thing about Jonathan's job is that he brings hot food home every day, a Godsend for us here without electricity. Post-hurricane fare is reduced to food that doesn't require refrigeration, i.e. peanut butter, canned tuna and anything freeze-dried. One night Jonathan brings home a lukewarm hamburger and French fries packed in a Styrofoam box, and I sit upstairs in the dark to savor every bite – I think it's the best hamburger I've ever eaten.

The following day I venture out of my compound to visit Mom, taking the most direct route south on U.S. 1 to use the least amount of gas. Police in yellow vests direct traffic at every major intersection, reminding me of conductors leading orchestras without the transcendent music and in a different state of mind. I survey the ravaged landscape: branches cracked like broken appendages, twisted metal blown off rooftops, discarded sculptures everywhere. Trees have been yanked from the ground, their roots stretched like rubber bands, hanging on for life. Live electrical wires dangle from concrete poles. Every gas station is closed, and I wonder when they will reopen. I only have ¾-tank of fuel left. I take it all in, feeling oppressed and stagnant, like the thick air that surrounds me.

Due to the multitude of so many obstacles, it has taken me longer to get to the hospital. Anxious to hug my mom after a scary and stressful night, I see her in bed and call out, "Mom!"

She has color in her face and looks as comfortable as she can with tubes in her nose and an IV in her hand.

"Jenna Doll!"

Although her Alzheimer's has progressed, she always knows me. We hug each other, relieved.

My siblings and I have decided to move her to the facility in Ohio whose admissions director tells us that transferring her directly from the hospital will facilitate the process.

"How would you like to go back home to Ohio, Mom?"

She stares at me for a moment. I'm not sure that she understands. She looks so weak.

"Remember Ohio? It's autumn, and the leaves are glorious."

Her words are jumbled and sentences cryptic, but I always understand what she is trying to say. She wants to go home.

Many calls are made. I persuade the doctors to keep her in the hospital for as long as the transfer process will take, a few days after she was due to be discharged. I visit her every day for nearly a week. My craving for hot food and air conditioning is satisfied at the hospital whose cafeteria has become a haven for the neighboring community. Between Jonathan's restaurant and the hospital, we live in relative post-hurricane luxury.

Flight arrangements are made for October 27. This will be my mother's homecoming, and I want her to look like her former, dignified self. It's turning cold up there, and she doesn't have shoes. I retrieved her best clothes from the communal grab bag at the Center, but must purchase her a nightgown, undershirts, shoes and socks. She needs to be warm. Another blessing, along with the hospital cafeteria, is Dadeland Mall which, thankfully, always opens soon after a hurricane.

The mall's parking lot is more crowded than I anticipated. People are restless, in need of air conditioning, hot food and stimulation. I want to conserve my cash because no power means no ATMs, but I can use my credit card at Macy's. As I look around I can tell who does and doesn't have electricity by the condition of their hair; greasy hair is a dead giveaway. I no longer feel self-conscious about mine.

I find Mom a floral flannel nightgown, cotton ankle socks and undershirts, enough layers to keep her warm. The clerk and I share hurricane tales, wishing each other good luck. I return to the first floor and find her a pair of navy Etienne Aigner leather flats, the kind she wore before being reduced to wearing slippers.

My next stop is to a pharmacy to fill the many prescriptions in my purse. I find one open and walk to the back of the store. Most of its lights are off, and no one else is around.

"Are you open?" I ask a man in a white jacket conversing with two co-workers. He glares and nods tentatively. "I have these prescriptions for my 91-year-old mother that need to be filled immediately."

I hand the prescriptions over to this stranger, trusting that he'll help me. He studies them and shakes his head. "We will have to order some, but they won't be here until tomorrow."

"You don't understand. I need them right away. We're leaving tomorrow morning. Isn't there something you can do?"

He doesn't apologize, but simply shakes his head, handing the papers back to me. I stand speechless, glaring at him with clenched fists.

I pull out of the parking lot and hope the CVS in my neighborhood might be open. They're usually accommodating, I say to myself as I continue to drive north. Some traffic lights are now working, so it doesn't take as long. I've made the trek south to see Mom for several days and notice my gauge now shows only ¼-tank of gas. I need enough to drive to the hospital tomorrow, then to the airport.

I'm in luck with the prescriptions and insist on waiting for the hour it will take to fill them all. I walk to my car to sit it out. A nearby Citgo station has reopened, and the scene is riotous: cars are lined up for blocks, police standing guard to maintain control and prevent irate customers from cutting in line. I watch screaming, honking, enraged sweaty men in t-shirts waving fists and cursing. I can't be a part of that. I convince myself that we'll get to the airport on fumes if necessary.

While waiting in my car, I call the travel agent to confirm my reservation. She listens to my hurricane and hospital tales and encourages me. I jot down confirmation numbers and special instructions for our Atlanta transfer.

Mom's prescriptions are now ready, and I add Ensure, apple juice, snacks and wet wipes for our flight, reminiscent of my travels with Jonathan when he was a child.

That evening I pack by candlelight; one bag for me, another for my mother. I can't see well but tell myself it doesn't really matter what I look like because I'm on a mission. My sisters will understand if nothing matches. The tension gripping my neck begins to ease under the soft glow of candlelight. I become aware of my shallow breath and consciously deepen it.

My mother's best clothes hang in my closet. I fold these into the suitcase, family photos tucked in between. All that is left of 91 years of living fits into this single suitcase. The enormous relief I feel, a sense that I am saving her, minimizes any sensation of sadness. I remove her travel outfit from the closet and place it in a plastic Publix bag. New socks, navy flats, Chico's pants and a cream-colored silk sweater that I'd hand-washed before the hurricane. I brace myself for a cold shower and wash my hair. It takes only 30 seconds; I'm clean enough.

When there's no electricity, bedtime is whenever the sun goes down. No TV, no reading without straining one's eyes, no entertainment to stretch out the evening. We leave the sliding glass doors and windows open for air, which compromises our sense of security. Sounds of the city – speeding cars, buses screeching to a stop and the abrupt wailing of police sirens – are silenced, thanks to the closed-off streets and power outages. Nature sounds prevail: rustling leaves, clucking cicadas and stillness. Sleep is elusive. My mind fills with "what if" anxieties about our journey tomorrow.

I rise with the sun and dress quickly. Breakfast consists of a banana and bottle of water. No power means no elevator. Jonathan and I lift and shove the suitcases with our knees, step by step, into the blackness of the underground garage. I consider our garage as a small blessing during hurricanes; no flying debris to damage our cars. We find our way in the dark, stuff one bag in the trunk and the other in the back seat, then head to the hospital, taking note of the gas gauge. I say a little prayer.

The drive is uneventful. Time is limited. We have to catch an 11:30 a.m. flight, and it's already 8. I turn into the hospital lot and park near the visitors' entrance. We head directly to the nurses' station to see if discharge papers have been processed.

"Hi. I'm Ivy Blackmore's daughter. We have an 11:30 a.m. flight to catch. She needs to be discharged as soon as possible."

"We're waiting for the doctor," says a nurse I don't recognize and who, apparently, doesn't appreciate the urgency.

I respond to her slowly, as though she were a small child, my voice a decibel lower than normal.

"I informed the nurse and social worker yesterday about our plans. They assured me everything would be in order."

She stares at me, unflinching, and in an irritated tone replies, "The doctor should start his rounds soon."

Her indifference infuriates me. I'm on speed and everything around me seems to be in slow motion. I search for the social worker involved in the transfer and see her at the end of the hall.

"Thank God you're here! Our plane leaves at 11:30. Where's the doctor? Can you can speed things up?"

I don't understand how they can be so lackadaisical – isn't *my* problem *their* problem? Her eyes give away her annoyance, but her voice is steady and unemotional.

"I'll try to see where he is."

She walks to the nurses' station and talks to the others on duty. I can see that I'm not winning any popularity contest.

I check on my mother who is sitting peacefully, hooked up to an IV and an oxygen machine. An aide is feeding her. She smiles, always happy to see me.

"Hi, Mom." I kiss her on the cheek. "We're going home today."

I charge ahead and ask the aide to help me dress her in her travel clothes while Jonathan goes to check the status of the situation. As I begin to take off my mother's hospital gown, the aide stops me.

"Wait a minute. The nurse needs to pull the IV first." She walks out to summon the nurse. The nurse and aide proceed to get Mom ready. Everything creeps forward as I take deep breaths to maintain my composure. She's finally dressed, discharge papers signed and the doctor has written a clearance letter for the airlines stating that Ivy is sufficiently stable to fly. We wheel her to the car, and I exhale. Jonathan has put her favorite Frank Sinatra CD on the car stereo. Soon, *I've Got the World on a String* and *Someone to Watch Over Me* fill the air.

"It's Frankie, Mom. He's your favorite."

I look at her next to me, dressed in her best travel clothes, looking like a delicate baby bird stunned and displaced from its nest, but trusting things will work out. A small smile emerges between tired breaths. She coughs in that all too-familiar way – wet, deep and from an unknown place in her lungs that frightens me. I pray she'll survive the day. She pulls up her silk sweater I lovingly hand-washed days earlier and wipes the phlegm from her mouth on it. I grab a wet-wipe from the door's side pocket and try to clean her with my right hand, holding the steering wheel with my left.

My thoughts flicker back and forth: *This is her homecoming; I want her to look elegant. After all, I've taken good care of her. No, it's more important that she arrive safely and in one piece. Don't worry about her clothes.* I glance at the gas gauge and see the red light flashing.

We pull up to the Delta terminal. Jonathan unloads the suitcases from the trunk as I approach the porter.

"Our plane leaves in 45 minutes, and my mother needs a wheelchair. Please help us." I notice my pressured speech as it erupts from my mouth, a clenched fist ready for battle.

He studies the tickets, photo IDs and my mother.

"Can she walk at all?"

"Not without help."

He turns to retrieve a wheelchair. Jonathan and I lift her gently and set her in it.

"The plane leaves from Gate D-9. Boarding begins in twenty minutes." He hands me our boarding passes and, looking at me with kind eyes, says, "Good luck."

"Thank you so much."

Jonathan stoops in front of his grandmother, his tall frame towering over her frail body.

"Bye, Grandma."

"Ooh, that feels good," she says with a smile. She pats his arm and kisses him on the cheek.

I'm worried about his ride home.

"Go straight to the nearest gas station, Jonathan. I know there's one open on Southwest Eighth Street."

"Don't worry, Mom." He always has a steady, reassuring presence, no matter the circumstance.

"I'll call you when we arrive."

We say our goodbyes, and I push my mother down the familiar, interminably long corridor to Gate D-9. I picked her up here some ten years ago, before 9/11, when we could still greet loved ones at the gate. Her breathing was labored even then, and we had to sit down every few minutes en route to the baggage claim. When my father was alive, the three of us joked about their staggering down to Florida from Ohio in mid-winter, never a moment too soon.

Gate D-9 is a beacon of light. I pull Ivy next to a chair and sit.

"We're here, Mom. We're going home. Are you hungry?"

She smiles and nods.

I dig into my bag filled with such essentials as her inhalers, juice, Ensure and applesauce. I pull out a strawberry Ensure and begin to feed her. I think about how long ago the aides at the Center started feeding her and wonder how it came to this and if she deliberately withdrew into herself, shut down because of the sickness, ugliness and chaos around her. I bury the thought. Not now; I'm on a mission.

Early boarding is announced, and I remind the agents that my mother can't walk by herself and requires assistance. I wheel her to the door of the aircraft where she's hoisted from her wheelchair into a special chair that fits in the narrow aisle. She winces.

"Please be careful!"

"It's okay, Mom."

We place her in a window seat. I take two blankets from the overhead bin and cover her. We sit side-by-side holding hands, her head resting on my shoulder. I think about the miraculous series of events that fell into place to make this moment happen: Mom's breathing problems that put her in the hospital during the hurricane, the social worker at the hospital who went out of her way to expedite the transfer, the administrator at the facility in Ohio who made it happen. And I never ran out of gas. It's meant to be. You're going home, Mom.

Full Circle

More than two years have passed since I took Ivy to Ohio. She's content in her new home. Everyone loves her. Unlike so many Alzheimer's patients whose personalities recede and disappear into a dark, unknown place, her sweet, beautiful spirit brightens as her dementia progresses. She's eternally grateful for everything and never fails to say, "I thank you," for even the smallest gesture. This hasn't gone unnoticed by her caregivers.

Jonathan and I visited her at both Thanksgiving and Christmas this last year, and she still recognizes us. She needs help walking, but is connected to her surroundings and still feeds herself. The nurses say she's at the beginning-of-the-end stage of Alzheimer's disease. I asked because I wanted to know, though it doesn't really matter now.

Ivy lives in a skilled nursing facility within walking distance of my sister Peggy's home. I visited every day when I came to Ohio for the holidays. This neighborhood is an older, more affluent community on the edge of the city. Ivy's home is at the bottom of a hill; its grounds punctuated with red maple, pin oak and evergreen trees. A narrow stream meanders along one side.

It's Christmas 2007, especially cold for Ohio, and Peggy and Annie walk with me to visit our mother. A Miamian now for so many years, I'm not used to temperatures below 50 degrees. Reinforced with multiple layers under Peggy's long, hooded woolen coat, I can see my breath on every exhale. We pass stately homes situated on large lots, flanked by century-old trees. It's easier walking down the hill.

"It's *really* cold."

"Your blood has thinned since you moved to Florida." Annie reminds me of this whenever I visit during the winter.

"Pick up the pace a little," says Peggy, who likes to give orders. Annie and I tease her, calling our attorney sister "the director."

I'm always tagging behind my sisters, an inclination since childhood. I prefer strolling to racing. My mind is elsewhere while walking, preoccupied with shapes and colors, nature's delicate patterns, memories evoked. I was never in a hurry to catch the school bus, though I liked school. But I'm making more of an effort today; it's Christmas, and I'm on my way to see Mom. But it's *freezing*.

We pass a wooden bridge spanning a narrow stream that flows beneath white patches of ice. Festive Christmas lights dot the compound of brick structures where Ivy now lives. After passing a large concrete planter filled with both blood red and creamy white poinsettias, we enter the building and I feel a blast of warm air. The thermostat must be set at about 85 degrees.

An addition was completed during this past year, and it's a longer walk to Mom's wing. A large Christmas tree is decorated with mittens of assorted sizes and colors. I notice the picture window where Ivy loves to sit. Outside there's a cylindrical bird feeder suspended from a maple tree and, in the immediate distance, a verdant expanse is sprinkled with tall evergreens. Squirrels, cardinals, robins and other of nature's treasures frequent this spot. Alongside the window is an illustrated guide to North American birds. Mom enjoys sitting here in her wheelchair, watching the show.

To the right is a dining room with a black upright Yamaha piano where several residents lounge in upholstered chairs.

My sisters and I brought our mother here for Thanksgiving, and I played some favorite tunes from our repertoire: *Rhapsody in Blue, Fascinatin' Rhythm, The Man I Love, Jesu Joy of Man's Desiring* and *Summertime* - Ivy used to play the counter-melody of this particular song during our duets.

When I started to play *Rachmaninoff's Prelude in D,* she started to cry. I had learned this in college and play it often – she loves it and is proud of me for mastering it. I continued to play, tears streaming down my face, knowing there will be no more duets and this tender moment may be our final songfest.

We reach the Alzheimer's wing whose residents are eating their Christmas lunch. Ivy is sitting at the table, and we sit next to her.

"Merry Christmas, Mom!"

We shower her with hugs and kisses. She smiles, glowing as always.

Christmas dinner is a soft rendition of prime rib, mashed potatoes, cranberry sauce, a green vegetable, a croissant and an apple cobbler. Ivy always eats her dessert first. We sit with her while she eats, cleaning her hands and mouth, picking up dropped morsels and handing her the milk carton and water.

Later we accompany her to a sitting room where two wing chairs upholstered in a satin floral pattern face its hearth. We pull up side chairs and the four of us sit facing the fire, like old times, happy. We stare for a few moments at flames crackling and spitting sparks, and Mom begins her speech.

"There's going to be a tairn, or torn. I think we are having a paraform."

She speaks with the authority of a wise mother imparting advice to her three daughters. For at least 20 minutes she gives an impassioned, loving, intimate speech, pausing on occasion, gesturing with her hands, laughing with us, listening as we respond, nodding her head in agreement and making her points.

It doesn't matter that her words are jumbled and nonsensical. We connect; we communicate.

She begins to tire, and we wheel her back to her room, passing the registration desk, the picture window with the bird feeder, open doors with residents visiting with family or watching television. The vertical photo album I assembled hangs from the ceiling to the top of her bed with smiling snapshots of family and friends spanning more than a half-century. We place her next to the CD player and put in her favorite Frank Sinatra disc. His smooth, sexy voice croons *Three Coins in a Fountain,* and Ivy closes her eyes and smiles. We hug and kiss her goodbye. My eyes always tear up whenever we part; I never know if this will be our last.

Pleasant Dreams

It's early June 2008, and I've once again made plans to visit Mom and my family in Ohio. My intuition tells me the end is near for my beloved mother; I'll stay a full month instead of my usual ten days. I'm staying for Mom's birthday; she'll be 94 on July 7.

I visit her soon after my arrival and am disheartened by obvious changes: her head droops lifelessly, as though her neck muscles have turned to rubber bands, and her hands twist inward, as it seems her soul is preparing for departure. The shades are drawn, shutters closed, portals sealed, and only a faint flicker of light remains. I feel sick inside.

I untwist her right hand and hold it tightly. As I nuzzle her cheek and kiss her, she leans her face into mine and smiles.

"It's Jenna, Mom. I love you."

"I love *you*."

Annie and I wheel her outside to the bench by the wooden bridge, where I recite her favorite passages of poetry. Her head is bowed, but I know she is listening. She adds the last word - "hair" of her favorite stanza from *The Highwayman*, and my sister and I sing *Twinkle Twinkle Little* Star and *Happy Birthday*.

I cup my hand on her cheek, and she whispers quietly, "Feeling the longing?" She's trying to tell me something.

Our visit is short; she seems so tired. We return her to the dining room. I lean over to kiss her goodbye.

A bebop song plays on the CD. Her head bowed, Ivy's shoulders sway to the music. She always loves a party.

I continue to visit daily and, as one visit ends, she whispers in my ear, "Not long."

Ten days later we're called and told that she's not expected to last the night. I race with my sisters, sister-in-law and our childhood friend to her bedside. She looks peaceful and beautiful, her silken-white hair freshly brushed and wavy. Oxygen tubes are in her nostrils. I curl up at the end of her bed and hold her hand as my tapes of our piano duets and favorite poetry are played. She smiles with tears in her eyes when she hears *Summertime* on the CD player. Tears stream down my face, too.

Annie and I spend the night. I rub my mother's legs, kiss and hug her, while my sister sits upright in the chair and watches her breathe. During one brief moment Ivy kisses my cheek and winks at me, like old times.

The nurses and aides, compassionate and solicitous, have set up a table with snacks and drinks. Our mother is so loved here. I watch as residents stroll by the table, studying the display like contents from a candy counter, taking whatever they please. A well-dressed gentleman, seemingly in charge, shows us to a room with a couch. Initially I think he is a staff physician making his rounds, but soon realize he's a resident and it's 3 a.m. A sweet lady with vulnerable, childlike eyes joins our vigil. I feel loved and cared for, as Mom must feel, too.

Ivy's roommate, an alto, sings in her sleep. I imagine her as a teenager, singing in the high school choir. A bright red-orange and blue-green floral still life painted by Mom's college friend hangs alongside her bed, a happy memory.

Sounds from an oxygen machine accompany our deathwatch, droning throughout the night, a dirge in a minor key that ends with a short melody and a sound akin to crashing cymbals...playing over and over and over again. The air feels so heavy.

Annie leaves at 7 a.m., while I remain until Peggy arrives an hour or so later. On my way home I see a poster announcing an upcoming walkathon to fund Alzheimer's research on June 28. I eat, shower and then return to Mom's bedside to resume the vigil. My sisters and I decide on three-hour shifts.

We talk to the doctor who confirms that the dying process has begun. We want her to be as comfortable as possible. He shuts off the oxygen machine, assuring us that as her organs shut down, she'll suffer no pain. I play Billie Holiday on the CD player.

"That's beautiful," she says with her eyes closed.

We moisten her lips with water from a sponge. She sometimes sucks on it, but gradually loses interest as her breathing becomes shallow. She curls up in a ball and feels cold. I kiss her and put on the soundtrack from one of our favorite movies, *Shine*. We rub and hug her, as her head moves back and forth rhythmically. Distressed, she cries out, "I don't know which way to go! Heaven!"

She calls out our father's name – "Robert!"

She writhes and moans as though trying to give birth, her head thrashing from side to side. It looks as if her soul is working its way through her body. Tears burn my eyes and my throat tightens, but I try to keep my composure.

After being given a small amount of morphine, Mom sleeps. Her doctor and nurses say she may last two or three more days but, of course, no one knows for sure.

I'm beginning to think she may want to be alone when she passes on; our presence may be distressing. She was always a private person. Maybe she wants to protect us.

I tell this to my sisters, and they agree. It's the afternoon of June 25, and we kiss our mother goodbye, then leave.

The next morning we get a call that our beautiful mother left us peacefully at 8:45 a.m. We hurry to her side and kiss her. I rub her legs like I did when I slept at the end of her bed for two nights. She is cold and stiff, but I'm relieved she is free. No more longing, no more yearning, no more pain.

Three weeks later, after returning to Miami, I seek some reassurance that my mother is "okay," so I contact a spiritual channeler who makes contact with my mother:

"I'm glad to be rid of that body and that mind," Mom says, joyful now that she's reunited with friends, family and our father. She wouldn't want to be anywhere else. My mother reassures me that, though moaning at the end might have made it appear she was suffering, she wasn't. Her soul was already transitioning.

"I love you very much. Thank you for taking care of me."

I asked if she forgave me for putting her in that facility in Miami.

"There's no reason for forgiveness, because you didn't do anything wrong. You had no choice. I know you did it out of love. By that time, it didn't really matter where I was. It didn't matter."

She was thankful to relieve my burden so I might get my life back in order.

"You're a good daughter and I'm proud of you. I thank you."

The pastor read Ivy's favorite stanza from *Thanatopsis* at her memorial service. This is the poem by William

Cullen Bryant she struggled to remember at the onset of her Alzheimer's.

So live, that when thy summons comes to join
The innumerable caravan, which moves
To that mysterious realm, where each shall take
His chamber in the silent halls of death,
Thou go not, like the quarry-slave at night,
Scourged to his dungeon, but, sustained and soothed
By an unfaltering trust, approach thy grave
Like one who wraps the drapery of his couch
About him, and lies down to pleasant dreams.

Pleasant dreams, my dear, sweet, beautiful mother.

A Beautiful Ending

It's June 9, 2009 and I'm back in Ohio for my annual visit. Mom's ashes still sit in a container on a shelf in Peggy's closet next to Dad's, who died some 13 years ago last February. It's been almost a year since Mom passed away...time for closure.

Our childhood home is now a holistic healing center. My brother discovered this two years ago when he returned here to watch his daughter's tennis matches at nearby Ohio State University. Walking around inside was a black cocker spaniel similar to one our family owned when we lived there. My sisters, brother and I decide this will be a perfect place to spread our parents' ashes.

I Google the address and several names come up: a massage therapist and two naturopathic doctors, as well as Susan, a psychic and metaphysical instructor. I call Susan who provides the name of the present-day proprietor of this property, a family compound for three generations. We're told the best way to contact the owner is to go to her house, which is located on the lot where our uncle, aunt and cousins had lived.

We drive there and knock on her door and a middle-aged woman with short curly blond hair and clear blue eyes comes to the door.

"Are you Alison?"

"Yes."

"Susan, the psychic who rents space at the house in back, told us we could find you here."

"Our parents built that house in 1950. They passed away, and we'd like to spread their ashes there. We have many happy memories," Peggy explains.

"Sure," responds the owner without hesitation. "That'll be fine. The house has such positive energy."

"We thought Sunday might be a good day, and we wouldn't bother anybody."

"Fine. Just drive on up and take your time," Alison says with a compassionate smile.

"Thank you so much. We really appreciate it," I add.

"I'm happy to accommodate you."

Sunday, June 14, my siblings and I arrange to meet in the afternoon. As my sisters, niece, nephew and I wind our way up the driveway we see our brother Bobby and his family exploring the neighboring woods. It seems like old times; exploring was a favorite pastime for all four of us. I hear the creek flowing over the rocks, calming my nerves. Our house looks the same, except that it's now blue, not green.

I carry the containers with our parents' ashes in a paper bag with a handle. It's heavy.

The others wait on a bridge that connects our property to a neighbor who, when we lived here, was a close family friend. Auntie Harpster was an elegant lady who never married and loved us as if we were her own. She had a thick white rug and a concert grand piano in her living room. My sisters and I joined her for tea parties and, next to our plates, were ceramic animal figurines she'd purchased lovingly for each of us. We accumulated a collection of horses, cats and dogs, later displaying them on a shelf by our beds.

After a heavy snowfall we would sled down her hill, bundled in long underwear, corduroy pants, wool sweaters and knitted hats that covered everything but our faces. We wore mittens and fur-topped, white rubber boots with buttons and hooks to make them snug. We marched across the creek and plodded up the big hill that, at our ages, looked more like a mountain. Some afternoons when it was freezing cold and the snow was wet and icy as a snow cone, we flew down the hill at lightning speed – sometimes into the frozen creek below. I loved the out-of-control feeling that I felt on our round, silver saucer-shaped sled.

The new house, more modern and expansive, sits on the hill. Alison's elderly parents are now living here.

I feel eight years old again, as though I had never left, and my last 48 years have been a flash of light, like the heat lightning I remember on warm summer evenings. As I again stand in this idyllic pastoral setting, I feel embraced by love, by family, memories and the security of a timeless, healing place that is, in spirit, my home.

My arm is tiring from the weight of the ashes, so I hand the bag to Peggy.

"I brought the Prayer of St. Francis of Assisi to read," says my nephew Gunner.

All ten of us stand together on the bridge and hold hands while he reads:

Lord, make me an instrument of your peace.
Where there is hatred, let me sow love;
Where there is injury, pardon;
Where there is doubt, faith;
Where there is despair, hope;
Where there is darkness, light;
And where there is sadness, joy.
O Divine Master, grant that I may not so much seek
To be consoled as to console;
To be understood as to understand;
To be loved as to love.
For it is in giving that we receive;
It is in pardoning that we are pardoned;
And it is in dying that we are born to eternal life.
Amen.

My eyes sting with tears, but I push them back.

We need to decide where to spread the ashes.

"This is the hard part," Bobby says.

"How about in the creek, where they would flow with the water?" I respond.

"But then they'll be gone," says Peggy.

We exchange sad smiles.

"Maybe around the Christmas tree?" Bobby suggests.

"Let's just spread them everywhere," I say. "And each of us can take a handful."

We agree. Peggy stands on the bridge holding Mom's ashes. I grab the bridge railing with my left hand, my hands and knees shaking as I step upon the uneven rocks that line the bank leading to the stream.

"Be careful!" Annie warns.

Bobby stands next to me with Dad's ashes. I reach in and scoop up a handful of Mom's, raise my arm high and thrust my hand over the stream, spreading my fingers wide to release their ashes into the flowing water. Finding more courage, I stand tall and resolute, and hurl a second handful into the stream.

Bobby does the same with Dad's.

They're both free, and so am I.

I feel a release of pent-up energy; my hands and knees no longer tremble.

Everyone joins in as we all walk around the grounds to spread the remaining ashes about the grounds.

"Let's spread some by the Buckeye tree. I remember falling out of it and having the wind knocked out of me," Peggy says.

"Let's put some by their bedroom," Bobby suggests.

We walk around the yard alongside the woods, spreading more.

"Remember when we made up names for the different parts of these woods?" I ask Peggy.

There once was an apple orchard adjacent to one side of the yard, later a pasture for the neighbor's horses. Now it's the rear of a shopping mall, trees buffering the view.

"I remember riding horses bareback here when no one was around until Mom had to rein me in," I recall.

We spread more ashes by Bobby's room.

"Remember your Superman comics?" I ask.

"And ships – the Nina, Pinta and Santa Maria," adds Annie.

We pass the room shared by Peggy and me.

"This is where those Martians, Indians and lions came at night," I say.

"I saw the lion by the stream," Peggy adds.

"He sniffed the end of your bed, too," I respond.

"I dreamed that hobos from the train had found us," Annie says.

We combine Mom's and Dad's ashes in one container and continue to the front of the house where we spread these next to their bedroom, then proceed toward the Christmas tree.

"I dug the hole to plant that one," Bobby says.

"You must have done a good job because it's thriving," I note.

An hour passes and we end at the red-bricked patio next to small Buddha and angel statues that border the steps. Everyone is smiling and laughing, reminded of heartwarming childhood memories and filled with a sense of peace. I know Mom and Dad are smiling.

The next afternoon I return to meet with the psychic I initially contacted, thankful to be able to see the interior of the house. As with the exterior, little has changed: a soft light filters through tall picture windows that flank the living room, now a reception area. Where our concert grand piano held sway, there are now a desk and file cabinets.

"I'm here to see Susan," I tell the receptionist.

"I'll tell her you're here."

All these furnishings are sleek, modern and tasteful, the same as when we lived here. I sit in one of the two blue chairs and, as my hands rest on its arms, a surge of energy pulses through me. I'm completely at ease, as though this were still my home and these healing practitioners my guests, called upon to perform their sacred work.

The proprietor sits at the desk closest to me and talks on the phone. I didn't realize she worked here as well, but notice she introduces herself as "Doctor." During a pause I address her.

"I met you two days ago. Thank you so much for allowing us to spread our parents' ashes here yesterday. It meant so much to us all."

"I'm happy for you. This is a special place. By the way, are you and your sisters triplets?"

I laugh and tell her no, but we look so alike that one of us is often mistaken for another.

My meeting with Susan is in Annie's old bedroom. I tell her that nothing has really changed since we lived here.

"The house doesn't need change. It's perfect the way it is."

She comments about the positive energy here and informs me that we are on a line of sacred Indian burial grounds. I didn't know this but am not surprised.

"Your Mom and Dad were with you yesterday. They're so grateful and appreciate the love you all put into it."

I feel the embrace of a soft light as she speaks.

We end the session and, as I step onto the patio, I notice some of Mom's and Dad's ashes on leaves outside the front door. I rub my hand over them, and then place them over my heart.

A sense of peace washes over me. I know Mom and Dad are with me in spirit – and for that I will be forever grateful.

Acknowledgements

I greatly appreciate my sisters Ann and Peggy Blackmore for both cheering me on and also for clarifying details of our shared childhood experiences.

I also thank Carol Williams, Elaine Schiffman and Diane Losada-Campos – long-time friends – and Susan Wagner, an International Women's Writing Guild colleague, for their support, encouragement and constructive criticism, as well as Judith Searle for her editorial assistance. Lastly, with heartfelt appreciation, I thank another dear friend, Al Alschuler, for sharing his professional expertise and for guiding me, lovingly, through the final stages of this project.